# WHEN WE DO HARM

# WHEN WE DO HARM

*A Doctor Confronts*
*Medical Error*

Danielle Ofri, MD

BEACON PRESS
BOSTON

BEACON PRESS
Boston, Massachusetts
www.beacon.org

Beacon Press books
are published under the auspices of
the Unitarian Universalist Association of Congregations.

23 22 21 20     8 7 6 5 4 3 2 1

This book is printed on acid-free paper that meets the uncoated paper
ANSI/NISO specifications for permanence as revised in 1992.

Text design and composition by Kim Arney

Names and identities of patients and their families have been changed,
unless permission was explicitly granted. The names of the medical
staff and the children in Jay's story are pseudonyms.

Several brief sections of this book originally appeared in the *New England
Journal of Medicine*, the *New York Times*, *Slate*, and the *Lancet*.

Library of Congress Cataloging number 2019051595
Library of Congress Cataloging-in-Publication Data is on file.

For Naava, Noah, and Ariel

*It may seem a strange principle to enunciate as the very first requirement in a hospital that it should do the sick no harm.*

*It is quite necessary, nevertheless, to lay down such a principle.*

—FLORENCE NIGHTINGALE, 1863

# CONTENTS

# JUMBO JETS CRASHING

"**I**s this *really* true?" my editor at Beacon Press emailed me skeptically. It was a spring afternoon in 2016 and she had tacked on an article from the *British Medical Journal* (*BMJ*) that caused headlines in the mainstream media (though it stirred up a healthy dose of criticism in academic circles).[1] Medical error, the article concluded, was the third-leading cause of death in the United States.

I floundered for an answer to her question, and not just because I hadn't been keeping up with the medical journals that pile up relentlessly in my clinic, in my mailbox, in my inbox, and, okay, even in my bathroom.

I floundered because I genuinely could not answer her question. Third-leading cause of death? *Really?* Did medical error really beat out breast cancer, stroke, Alzheimer's disease, accidents, diabetes, and pneumonia?

As a practicing internist for the past twenty-five years at Bellevue Hospital, one of the largest and busiest hospitals in the United States, I feel as though I see a reasonable cross-section of medicine today. My patients suffer overwhelmingly from the ailments of a twenty-first-century "developed" society—obesity, diabetes, heart disease, hypertension, cancer.

If medical error is the third-leading cause of death, then I should be seeing it all the time, right? I should be hearing about it from friends and family. If medical error clocks in just after heart disease and cancer as a killer, it should be part of my everyday medical experience.

But it isn't.

Or at least it doesn't feel that way.

I have witnessed medical errors, of course, and I've certainly made my share of them. I've heard bone-chilling tales in hospital corridors and read shocking, heart-wrenching stories in the media. Yet these all feel like exceptions—

rare and horrible. These deaths don't pop up in my clinical practice with a frequency remotely near that of congestive heart failure, lung cancer, or emphysema.

Yet the data keep coming. From the first Institute of Medicine report in 1999[2] that estimated 44,000 to 98,000 deaths per year from medical error to this *BMJ* analysis suggesting upward of 250,000 deaths per year—medical error seems on the verge of a public health emergency. Even if the numbers aren't completely precise—the methodologies of these papers have been challenged—researchers are in agreement that the number of errors is not small at all.

Are the data wrong? Or am I wrong?

Am I—and most medical staff—simply not seeing this epidemic? Are we biased? In denial? Are we clinicians killing our patients at an unprecedented rate and somehow remaining blithely unaware? If that's really the case, perhaps we should take down our collective shingles and spare our patients the damage. We could just tack a note onto the door: "Eat quinoa and beans. Take the stairs. Stay away from the healthcare system."

While the "third leading cause of death" claim is likely an overstatement, there is definitely a yawning gap between the published statistics of medical error and the experience of the everyday clinician. And then there are the experiences of the everyday patient, which also diverge from the data but in different ways.

As a practicing physician—and an occasional patient myself—I feel I have to get to the bottom of this. What I experience and what the published data conjecture seem at complete odds. One of us is calling it wrong, and my goal is to find out who.

---

If the history of medicine over the past two hundred years were a feature film, it would be a swashbuckling adventure epic. Heroes in white coats would brandish stethoscopes and pipettes, decapitating disease in single fell swoops with their medical machetes. Sanitation, antisepsis, and anesthesia would hurl across the screen, flattening 19th-century illnesses. Vaccines and antibiotics would explode like grenades in the early 20th century—rescuing the masses from infectious marauders. Our triumphant superheroes would swagger into the second half of the twentieth century, whirling about to execute 360 degrees of jujitsu strikes—chemotherapy, dialysis, antipsychotics, blood transfusions, birth control, CT scanners, cardiac catheterization, ICUs, statins, antihypertensives, HIV treatment—slaying every dragon in the room with hardly a backward glance. The movie would be one straight trajectory of progressive victory over disease, nearly doubling average life expectancy before you even approached the unpopped kernels at the bottom of your greasy popcorn box.

Staggering success has been the dominant leitmotif in medicine. With good reason! Turning once-uniform killers into afterthoughts is an impressive feat that should not be taken for granted. But this theme of relentless victory hasn't left much space in the narrative for talking about the medical errors and adverse outcomes of our treatments. At best, these were annoying pebbles along the road upon which our heroes confidently strode.

It's not that medicine does not examine errors. Morbidity and mortality conferences—affectionately known as M&Ms—have been a part of medicine for a century. M&Ms were, and still are, formal evaluations of bad outcomes. But the rugged individualism of our medical heroes filtered through to our analysis of medical mistakes, with the general approach being to figure out what—or more often *who*—had malfunctioned and then fix that thing. Still, these errors were seen as mere footnotes to the inexorable sense of progress. All would get fixed by the indefatigable advances of medical research.

It's not surprising, therefore, that the tallying of medical harms was never a flourishing area of medical research. The gray-haired establishment of medicine was of the view that the noble art of medicine—bolstered by the juggernaut of scientific research—was exemplary in its ministrations. Instead it was the trainees, in fact, who were among the earliest to point out the blind spots.

Robert Moser, a resident at Brooke Army Medical Center, was one of the first people to take a hard look at the downsides of medical care. In a 1956 paper in the *New England Journal of Medicine*, he described "diseases that would not have occurred if [the] therapeutic procedure had not been employed." This paper may have been the first to survey the damages that we clinicians do, even in the name of good medical care. He titled his paper "Diseases of Medical Progress" and found that about 5% of patients experienced these.[3]

A few years later, this paper happened to be discussed during a morning conference of the medical residents at Yale-New Haven Hospital. Among the residents present that day was Elihu Schimmel, whose main claim to academic fame thus far had been a gold medal in Talmud at the Eitz Chaim yeshiva of Borough Park, Brooklyn. Schimmel was struck by the uncomfortable idea that the medicine he was learning could cause harm as well do good. During his training he began keeping his own score card, noting any complications or poor outcomes he felt were the result of the medical treatments he was giving.

After three years of training, Schimmel was selected to be the chief medical resident for the 1960–61 academic year. It was a tradition at Yale that the chief resident undertake a research project, and Schimmel decided to expand on Moser's work. Moser had examined his cases retrospectively, and all retrospective analyses—like Monday morning quarterbacking—are fraught with bias. Schimmel wanted to be more scientifically rigorous and examine the problem *prospectively*. He would document, in real time, how many complications patients experienced as a result of their medical care. "This was the first study to produce both numerator *and* a denominator," Schimmel told me with pride.

The foot soldiers of the study would be the thirty-three residents who made up Yale's medical residency program. "It was clear that this would not fly on the surgical service," he recalled with a chuckle, sensing that the more buttoned-up Department of Surgery would not be keen to air its dirty laundry.

Starting on August 1, 1960, every chart of every patient had a form tacked onto the front of it. The medical residents were to note any untoward event, even if it occurred as a result of a necessary and acceptable treatment or test. Schimmel specifically excluded events that occurred as a result of an inadvertent error (e.g., accidentally grabbing the wrong medication). He was more interested in the harm that came from the medical care itself. The study went on for the next eight months and included just over a thousand patients.

The residents recorded 240 adverse events that occurred in 198 patients. That meant that about 20% of patients experienced some sort of harm as a result of their medical care. This was an astonishing number. No one in the medical field would have estimated that their actions would harm one of every five patients.

It turned out that in the Department of Dirty Laundry, the Department of Medicine was just as reticent as the Department of Surgery. None of the senior faculty in Schimmel's department offered to coauthor the paper— as would usually happen when a resident undertook a research project. So Schimmel wrote the paper solo.

Nor, it seemed, was the general medical field particularly keen on the public airing of dirty laundry. "We don't publish things like that at the *New England Journal of Medicine*," he was told. After numerous rejections, his 1964 paper was ultimately published in the *Annals of Internal Medicine*.[4]

Neither the topic of Schimmel's paper nor the title—"The Hazards of Hospitalization"—endeared him to many, especially at an Ivy League institution like Yale. He'd already rankled the upper crust a year earlier when he published a provocative commentary about iatrogenic illness—diseases caused by doctors.[5] (That article carried the deliciously skewering title "The Physician as Pathogen.") After Schimmel presented the results of his "Hazards of Hospitalization" study at Grand Rounds, the director of the hospital hauled him into his office. "What *is* this that you are saying about New Haven Hospital?" he demanded to know.

"There were no hazards involving the hospital *building*," Schimmel noted drily. "Hospitals don't practice medicine." The rest he left unsaid.

---

It was not until the 1980s that researchers began examining medical harms on a larger scale. The lens, though, was not really patient safety, a term that had not yet even been coined. Rather, it was the American malpractice system. Were doctors getting sued out of existence? Could patients win enough money to cover the spiraling costs of healthcare? What happened to the patients who couldn't get their day in court? These questions could not be answered because no one really knew the extent of the problem. How many patients were getting injured in the medical system? How severe were these injuries? Were these "side effects" of good medical care or bad outcomes related to outright negligence? What was the economic impact?

One of the first studies to examine these questions in a rigorous way was the Harvard Medical Practice Study.[6] The researchers studied fifty-one hospitals in the state of New York over the calendar year of 1984. (If dirty laundry was to be aired, presumably these Harvard researchers preferred it to be of New York origin, rather than from their own hospitals in Massachusetts!) They examined 30,121 randomly selected charts and recorded the number of adverse events, which they defined as unintended injuries resulting from medical care. The study found that 3.7% of hospitalizations resulted in a medical injury, of which 14% were fatal. If the study results were extrapolated to all residents of New York State, this would mean that there were nearly one hundred thousand injuries (including 13,451 deaths and 2,550 cases of permanent disability) as a result of hospital care in 1984.

One of the authors of the study, a pediatric surgeon named Lucian Leape, was so stunned by the magnitude of harm to patients that he hung up his scalpel and spent the rest of his career drilling into these data. He was particularly struck by the fact that some two-thirds of the injuries were felt to be potentially preventable. Moreover, the study had recorded only the errors that resulted in significant injury. There were undoubtedly far more errors that went unnoticed because the injuries were minor. And what about all the errors that hadn't caused harm? These were still errors and represented an even larger minefield of potential catastrophe.

Leape published a seminal article in 1994 that reoriented the focus of medical-error research away from the malpractice system toward the overall goal of making healthcare safer.[7] For starters, data collection needed to focus on the *total* number of errors, not just the ones that caused harm; medical professionals could not rest easy just because an error did not happen to leave the patient with an injury. Leape's primary theme, however, was that errors were usually the result of failures of *systems*, not just failures of individuals. Even if the proximate cause of an error was, in fact, a human action, such as a nurse administering the wrong medication, you could almost always uncover layers of systems errors that made the error possible.

In this example, it could be that the nurse was responsible for too many patients, or her train of thought was constantly interrupted by alarms, or the medications had sound-alike names, or the location of the medications was different on each ward, or the super-shiny label was impossible to read in the glare of fluorescent lights. Whereas hospitals would typically respond by disciplining the nurse or mandating remedial training, Leape's message was that if the hospital *really* wanted to prevent future errors, it would have to dig deeper into the system to figure out what had made the nurse's error possible. "Errors must be accepted as evidence of systems flaws," he wrote, "not character flaws."

The second theme Leape hammered home was that errors in medicine are inevitable. He described it as a fundamental mistake that healthcare systems "rely on individuals *not* to make errors rather than to assume they will." He was intrigued by cognitive psychology and the field of human factors research (engineering design that focuses on how humans and machines interact). By understanding how humans think and respond in certain situations, we could learn how and why we make many of the typical errors in medicine. Armed with that information, we could redesign the system to make it more difficult for people to make errors.

(The third "theme" from Leape's article was his observation that if the fatal injuries from the Harvard Medical Practice Study were extrapolated to the entire United States, it would be the equivalent of a jumbo jet—and a half!—crashing every single day. The demolished airplane thus became the defining metaphor of the nascent patient-safety movement.)

Leape was part of a group that authored the groundbreaking report *To Err Is Human* for the Institute of Medicine in 1999. Many people consider the IOM report to be the founding document of the modern patient-safety movement, talked of with the same reverential awe as the Dead Sea Scrolls or the US Constitution. *To Err Is Human* stressed that medicine needed to work more on making the system safer and less on blaming individual people for their errors. The IOM report was leaked to the media, and its estimate of up to 98,000 Americans dying each year as a result of medical error grabbed headlines. The jumbo jet metaphor was ubiquitous, with splashy pictures of plane crashes used wherever journalistically possible.

Contrary to popular conception, though, *To Err Is Human* was not a research study. No one donned a Sherlock Holmes cape and started snooping for fingerprints in emergency rooms. No one peeked into operating rooms or trailed nurses on rounds. No one pored through medical records or sat in on autopsy sessions. What the IOM report did was take the data from the Harvard Medical Practice Study (which, as a New Yorker, I feel duty-bound to point out should have been named the *New York* Medical Practice Study) and data from a similar study done in Utah and Colorado[8] and extrapolate these to the entire United States. The much quoted number of 98,000 deaths per year came from the mathematical exercise of considering New York to be the entire country (which, of course, we New Yorkers already know to be true). If the US consisted solely of sparsely populated rectangular states like Utah and Colorado, the annual death toll from medical error would be 48,000. So the official estimate of deaths due to medical error from the IOM report was a range of 48,000 to 98,000.

The lower number was quickly lost in the media frenzy. As was just about every other lick of nuance. All anyone could talk about was how doctors were killing off 98,000 Americans every year. One of the biggest facts ignored by the media was that the two main studies upon which the IOM report was based involved *hospitalized* patients. Most people do not get their medical care in hospitals, so already the data are not generalizable. Hospitalized patients are by definition sicker than the general population and usually older. Sicker patients have many more treatments, medications, and procedures, and interact with more medical personnel than the average person—a point I'll come back to several times in the book. Even if all of these are transacted with 99% perfection, the sheer number of moving parts that orbit a hospitalized patient nearly guarantees that there'll be at least one thing in the mix that doesn't go as planned.

The second nuance that was missed was the issue of preventability. The original studies did not set out to ascertain what percentage of errors were preventable—they were studying medical injuries and malpractice cases. When researchers went back later to extract that information, they had only case summaries to analyze, not the original medical charts. Much detail was lost, and the researchers themselves had trouble agreeing on which errors would be considered preventable.

Moreover, preventable *errors* and preventable *deaths* are two very different things. For example, a patient dying from end-stage liver disease might have been given an incorrect dose of an antibiotic. This, then, is a patient who experienced both a preventable error as well as a death, but these two things are not necessarily related. Fixing the antibiotic dose—i.e., preventing the error—would not have altered the death from liver disease. Figuring out whether an error actually *caused* a death requires intricate analysis. So yes,

98,000 people who died may have experienced an error during their medical treatment. But was it the error that cause their death? The IOM report could not answer that question, and the media could not be bothered with such parsings. The headline was just too juicy to pass up.

It is likely that we do *not* have a jumbo jet's worth of patients crashing on US soil every day as a result of our misdeeds. The number is probably smaller. However, it's not zero. Even if the 98,000 estimated deaths per year as a result of medical error are really 50,000 or 20,000 or 5,000, that's still way too many patients dying from our actions. Plus, *death* from medical error is only a tiny subset of the patients who are harmed by error. What about the patients who suffer bleeding or kidney failure or blood clots as a result of error? Those are significant harms, even if they don't result in death. Additionally, we are now coming to view misdiagnoses and delays in diagnosis as errors too, thus enlarging the tent of "preventable harm."

So while the IOM report may not have been fully accurate—and certainly the news media flushed away any subtlety of analysis—it succeeded in focusing the attention of both the medical field and the public on the issue of patient safety. It also got the grant-funding wheels rolling, allowing researchers to study medical error with the depth that we study other diseases that cause harm to humans. An original copy of *To Err Is Human* probably won't get you as much as an original copy of the Beatles' White Album, but it ultimately served its purpose of jump-starting the patient-safety movement.

---

Often in medicine we are told to "take a page" from the aviation industry. Given the state of modern airlines, I'm sure I'm not alone in hoping that we don't take the page on legroom or baggage fees, but there is definitely much to be learned from our airborne counterparts. The aviation industry started out like medicine, an open laboratory for rugged individualists, in this case adventurous mavericks battling gravity and physics. But a turning point occurred in 1935 in the now-famous tale of the B-17 "Flying Fortress" bomber. This was the most advanced aircraft of its day, developed to keep the US military the dominant fighting force in the world. It was bigger and faster than anything that had preceded it and sported the most sophisticated control systems ever seen in a cockpit. On its maiden voyage, however, it exploded within 30 seconds of takeoff. It was later determined that the pilot had neglected to disengage the locks on the moveable flaps of the wings known as control surfaces.

If this were a medical case, the pilot would be up on the stand in an M&M, shamefacedly recounting how he'd forgotten to unlock the control surfaces. The senior physicians fortifying the front row would gesticulate with their reading glasses as they elaborated on how immobilized control surfaces prevent a pilot from adjusting the pitch of the airplane. The plane would thus be cemented at a fixed angle, with the pilot unable to make adjustments. This would be akin to driving a car with wheels fixed in one direction, unable to turn.

On the stand, the pilot would remain stone still while the pathophysiology was painstakingly explicated and the inevitable path toward catastrophe laid out for all to see. His flagellation would be achieved without a word of chastisement even having to be uttered. Half the audience would be thinking, "What an imbecile," with the other half reaching for their rosaries and muttering, "Thank God it wasn't me in the cockpit."

That this did not happen was not just because the pilot had sadly perished in the explosion. It didn't happen because although human error was deemed the proximate cause of the crash, the error was *not* attributed to the pilot simply not being good enough. (As chief of flight testing for the entire US Army, this pilot possessed more expertise than most.) Rather, the diagnosis of human error was attributed to a system that had too many moving parts for one person to realistically attend to. This high-end jet had so many advanced and novel gizmos that the pilot simply couldn't keep track of them all. Sixty-five years before the IOM's *To Err Is Human*, the aviation industry made the decisive shift from focusing on individuals as the sources of error to focusing on systems that make errors possible.

From this experience, the aviation checklist was developed. The list has been adapted over the decades, but the ritual of the checklist endures. Some of the mystique of piloting a plane ebbed away with this more technician-like approach to flying. On the other hand, this more rigorous approach improved the safety of flight. The B-17 bomber, for example, never had an accident like that again. Overall, plane crashes and passenger deaths have steadily declined.

Periodically, the idea of a checklist for medicine popped up in various academic circles. It never got much traction because medicine was felt to be infinitely more complex than aviation. Doctors took umbrage at the very thought of checklists—they were not technicians like pilots! One could not checklist the alchemy of science, art, intuition, and bedside manner that created the greatest physicians.

It wasn't until 2001, just after the IOM report, that checklists had any sizable impact in medicine. Largely, this is because the developer—Peter Pronovost—did *not* attempt to checklist the complex alchemy of medicine. He chose to tackle one single concrete task—central lines—with the goal of eliminating one single adverse outcome—catheter-related infections.

Central lines are the large-bore catheters inserted into the major veins of the body—jugular, subclavian, femoral—when patients require prodigious amounts of fluids and medications, or have simply run out of smaller veins after extensive medical care. Patients who need them tend to be very sick and are often in the ICU. And if these catheters get infected, bacteria can quickly overwhelm these already compromised patients (as I'll describe in upcoming chapters with a patient named Jay). In the ICUs at Johns Hopkins Hospital, where Pronovost worked at the time, 11% of patients with central lines developed infections.

Pronovost's checklist seemed rather ridiculous—wash your hands, clean the patient's skin, cover the patient with a sterile drape, wear sterile garb, then put a sterile dressing on the patient when you are done. It was like he was checklisting the steps of brushing your teeth. Everyone knows how to brush your teeth—you do it automatically—so what good would a checklist do?

His experiment in the ICU has now assumed legendary status, because central-line infections essentially dropped to zero at his hospital.[9] And when the checklist was tried with nearly one hundred ICUs in seventy different hospitals in Michigan, infection rates also plummeted to near zero within three months.[10] It seemed almost too good to be true.

A similar checklist for the operating room was created by an international collaborative including Pronovost's colleague Martin Makary (one of the authors of the *BMJ* paper about errors as the third-leading cause of death) and Atul Gawande, a surgeon and medical writer from Boston. This one contained nineteen items, some as basic as introducing everyone on the team by name and role. There were the expected items—confirming the patient's name, type of surgery, and allergies; making sure IV fluids and blood transfusions were available; counting all the instruments and sponges before and after the surgery. And there were a few that required thought, such as outlining possible complications in advance. They tested it out in eight hospitals worldwide, from London and Seattle to Tanzania and India. Complication rates decreased from 11% to 7%, and death rates fell from 1.5% to 0.8%.[11]

Checklists garnered effusive news media coverage—here was a simple, low-tech intervention that would keep all those jumbo jets from dropping out of the sky—and quickly came to be seen as the answer to every patient-safety problem. After all, they'd apparently solved everything in aviation. From administrators' point of view, checklists were ideal—cheap, unambiguous, easy to initiate. All you had to do was distribute a sheet of paper to your staff. Hospitals began checklisting everything from preventing blood clots and treating strokes to discussing DNRs (do-not-resuscitate orders) and diagnosing brain death. You could hardly snag a snack from a hospital vending machine without encountering a checklist. And if administrators loved them, you could imagine how much government officials would love them.

In 2010, the Ministry of Health in Ontario mandated that all hospitals in the province use the surgical checklist. After all, if the Tanzanians could pull it off as well as the Londoners, it should be a cakewalk in rule-abiding Canada. Researchers gathered data before and after the implementation from nearly every hospital in the province, readying themselves to show the world how to improve medicine on a grand scale.

Well, it didn't quite turn out that way. Despite a 92–98% compliance rate with using the checklist, there wasn't a flicker of improvement. Mortality rates didn't budge. Complication rates stayed the same. No matter how the researchers sliced and diced the data—by age, by sex, by type of surgery, by acuity, by type of hospital—not one group did better after the checklist was instituted.[12]

How could that be? How could a checklist that worked equally well in teeming charity hospitals in New Delhi and swank university hospitals in Seattle not make a dent in sensible Ontario? The answer lies in the fact that we humans are enamored of catchy solutions (such as simple checklists) and are far less interested in the messy process of getting these things to work. Peter Pronovost would be the first to tell you that his piece of paper with five check boxes wasn't what eradicated the central-line infections. Eradicating the infections required a wholesale change in the culture of medicine, something that is arduous, tedious, decidedly un-newsworthy, and not universally welcomed in the medical sandbox.

The first thing Pronovost had to do when he began his project was to convince his colleagues that central-line infections were a preventable harm. This might seem ridiculously obvious now, but at the time most medical professionals thought of these infections as something that would occur inevitably in a certain percentage of cases. It was like a side effect of a medication, an unfortunate outcome that some patients experience, and you just had to balance this downside against the upside. Thinking of central-line infections as preventable harms required a major recalibration of mind-set.

The second thing he had to do was convince people to actually *measure* the infection rates. You'd think this was also a no-brainer, but many hospitals had no idea of the magnitude (or location) of the problem.

The third, and likely most important, part was that the rules of communication had to change. It certainly wasn't that checklists brought any breaking news to the table. I mean, every doctor *knows* you have to wash your hands before you insert a central line. Every surgeon *knows* you have to have IV fluids accessible before you start an operation. But by making these explicit on the checklist, the members of the team had to actually talk about it. The real hurdle—and what might ultimately be considered the secret sauce of Pronovost's original checklist—was that nurses were empowered to speak up.

This was a culture shift of epic proportions. It's not that nurses were docile sheep of 1950s vintage who were too afraid to make a peep about anything. It's more that in the grand scheme of things, with thousands of micro-decisions and micro-interactions every day, individual nurses always had to make a calculation about what was worth upsetting the apple cart over. Many doctors did not respond well to nurses chiding them about seemingly small annoyances such as washing hands. But nurses were the ones who could see what was happening on the ground and would potentially be the key to improving the situation.

However, it wasn't enough just to tell nurses that they had the right to speak up if a doctor didn't do all five steps. The real power was in getting the hospital administration to support them. Nurses were given the power to pull the plug on anything that didn't follow the correct procedure, and the suits in the boardroom promised to have their backs. In Pronovost's first trial at his own hospital, he told the nurses that they could page him, day or night, and he would personally back them up.

In an interview with the *New York Times*, Pronovost observed that "in every hospital . . . patients die because of hierarchy."[13] Anyone who works in healthcare has to take a step back and let that sobering statement sink in. It's not just nurses who find it difficult to speak up. Family members, medical students, clerical staff, nurse aides—these are all people who are lower on the medical totem pole and often don't feel comfortable contradicting senior doctors. But when it comes to preventing medical error, these are the folks on the front lines and are often the ones who see what's really happening. Bucking entrenched hierarchy, though, is not easy.

As a third-year medical student, I once assisted on a late-night operation when suddenly the surgeon's needle accidentally pricked my finger (I had been holding a liver or some random intestines out of the way). I couldn't tell from the eyes darting over the masks who else had noticed. I thought maybe the nurse had seen, but I couldn't be sure. Nobody said anything. The operation seemed to drag on for hours after that, and I spent the entire time frozen in my spot, debating whether and how I should say something. In the end, I couldn't muster the strength to push back against the hierarchy's deafening silence from my lowly perch as a medical student. That I left my wounded finger submerged in blood for the duration of the surgery during the height of the AIDS epidemic, and then was forced to agonize over repeated HIV tests in the weeks and months that followed, gives you an inkling of just how hard it is to speak up when the system expects you to shut up and not make trouble.

---

Lucian Leape, who is now often called the father of the patient-safety movement, wrote a thoughtful commentary after the Ontario ICU study rained on everyone's checklist parade. "The key," he said, "is recognizing that changing practice is not a technical problem that can be solved by ticking off boxes on a checklist but a social problem of human behavior and interaction."[14] When the focus becomes the checklist itself—as opposed to the people who are doing the actions—nothing will get accomplished. "Gaming is universal," wrote Leape, especially when checklists are mandated from the top down, as was the case in Ontario. The reported compliance rate of 92–98% is *diagnostic* of gaming, as we might say in medicine. A 98% compliance rate simply means that 98% of the time someone checked a box. That's all.

Which brings us to the real reason why some checklists work while others don't, or really why any intervention—to prevent medical error, to prevent disease, to improve health, to improve efficiency—works or doesn't work. It is all in how the intervention is actually accomplished on the ground, or what the technocrats call implementation. This is the boring aspect of medicine, not nearly as exciting as groundbreaking research or dramatic lifesaving interventions. These are the drab logistics of how to make the intervention happen: Where will the supplies be located? When exactly will the procedure be done? Will extra time be allotted for it? Who will be in charge of making sure it happens? Will someone explain to the staff why all these changes are happening? Who do you call if there's a problem? Who is going to be the champion and cheerleader for the change? What exactly should be measured to see if it's working? Is anyone going to get feedback on this? Has anyone thought about possible unintended consequences? Is anyone going to provide coffee?

The implementation list is long and extraordinarily detailed—it's a checklist in and of itself!—but if these issues aren't addressed, a checklist or any other intervention is doomed to fail. One morning in my clinic, as I was seeing my first patient of the day, I noticed that the electronic medical record (EMR) looked a little different. Apparently there had been some sort of "rollout" of various updates in the wee hours of the night, and now a bunch of minor things were out of order and tripping me up.

My fingers automatically knew, for example, that Spanish was #41 when it came to the language spoken by the patient, since Spanish is our most common second language. Knowing the number by heart saved me the aggravation of scrolling through the whole list. But somehow in this rollout, another language had been added, bumping Spanish to #42. My fingers still went to #41, though, so every patient that day came out speaking Serbian.

And then all of sudden, three brand-new fields popped up that I'd never seen before: latex allergies, food allergies, and environmental allergies. We'd always had a required allergies field, and you could enter any kind of allergy—medication allergies, food allergies—or even free-text other kinds of allergies (a few times I'd been tempted to write in "EMR allergy," but I restrained myself). But now these three new required fields popped up, and they each demanded my attention.

Now, it's not that I think latex, food, and environmental allergies are unimportant, but their inopportune debut made a hard day even harder. I typically type most of my notes after the patient has left the room, to avoid having the computer be the focus of a visit. So now I would encounter those new fields and face the prospect of sprinting out to flag down patients before they entered the elevator, hollering incoherently about latex gloves, kiwi fruits, and cat dander, smack in the middle of a day when everyone was suddenly speaking Serbian.

I recognized that these additional fields in the EMR were interventions to prevent medical error. They were placed there as part of a well-meaning effort on behalf of our patients to avoid using latex gloves if they were allergic or to make sure the staff didn't inadvertently deck the halls with boughs of ragweed during holiday season. But I found myself incensed by the whole process. The hospital was already using latex-free gloves, so the potential yield on that effort was distinctly low. But filling in these boxes took away time from focusing on things such as diabetes and heart disease that were really posing threats to my patients' safety.

You can be sure there was a 100% compliance rate on this effort—it was a required field, so no doctor could close out a note until something had been entered. Somewhere in some office there was a midlevel manager proudly reporting to his supervisor that the medical staff was "100% compliant." Did this effort actually advance the cause of patient safety in our hospital? I highly doubt it, since nearly everyone gave up in frustration and just clicked "no" to the latex allergy question (and faked the food and environmental allergy questions as well).

At the time I viewed this whole episode as just one more EMR annoyance and one more example of bumbling administration. But after reviewing the experience with checklists, I can see it as an implementation disaster. It was a laudable patient-safety intervention that lacked even the slightest attention to implementation. We had not been given any heads-up that we'd have to start asking patients about latex allergies or that our Hispanic patients would start yammering away in Serbian. No one thought through the unintended consequences of rejiggering the workflow that hundreds of doctors were doing automatically. No one thought about the time it would take. No one seemed to weigh the potential value of this intervention in a hospital that does not use latex gloves. (Yes, there are some latex catheters, but gloves are the overwhelming source of latex.) No one asked whether the juice was worth the squeeze.

This approach to allergies illustrates how checklists can become victims of their own success. Once you start checklisting everything, it devolves into checklist overload. One of the reasons the central-line and surgical checklists worked well was that they were the only checklists on the block. Once you have dozens in play, doctors and nurses can't cope. There are so many things to check off that you can hardly take care of your patients. Everyone just checks off everything to make it all go away. It's not necessarily a deliberate gaming of the system; it's a survival mechanism.

A number of lessons can be gleaned from these initial forays into decreasing medical error and improving patient safety. One is that you have to address the system as a whole; piecemeal efforts get you only so far. Another is that if you overemphasize "100% compliance," you will most certainly end up with people gaming the system, even if they aren't doing it with malicious intent. But really, the most crucial lessons are that if you don't focus on human behavior, how we mortals communicate, how the system works, and the all-important implementation, even the best solutions are doomed to fail. Of course, if any of us had read our history books, we would already have known that.

---

In the summer of 1846, a young Hungarian doctor named Ignaz Semmelweis was appointed to be the equivalent of the chief resident of the obstetrical service at Vienna General Hospital. The hospital had two maternity wards that were called, in typically utilitarian medical terminology, the First Clinic and the Second Clinic. The destitute of Vienna came to these clinics to deliver their babies because the medical care was free. The flip side of the deal was that these patients were part of a teaching service, attended to by trainees who were supervised by more senior staff. The First Clinic was the training site for medical students, and the Second Clinic was the training site for midwives.

For simplicity of scheduling, the two clinics alternated their admitting days. But Dr. Semmelweis quickly learned that patients vastly preferred the Second Clinic, and that they would do almost anything to be admitted to the

Second Clinic over the First Clinic. The reputation of the First Clinic was that it was the place where you went to die.

But it wasn't just reputation that made the First Clinic so undesirable—there were data to back this up. Puerperal fever (also known as childbed fever) was a rampant killer of otherwise healthy mothers at the time. The mortality rate in the First Clinic was vastly higher than in the Second Clinic, sometimes tenfold higher. Patients begged, wept, and pleaded to gain admittance to the Second Clinic. There were stories of women opting to give birth on the street rather than take their chances in the First Clinic.

As chief resident, Semmelweis was determined to figure out the reason for the striking difference in mortality rates. Because the wards admitted on alternate days, the patients were randomly distributed, at least in theory. In practice, though, the Second Clinic housed many more patients, because women did everything possible to get themselves admitted there. Even with that increased workload, mortality was still lower in the Second Clinic. Semmelweis examined every characteristic he could think of that might explain the mortality difference between the two clinics, including breastfeeding rates, religious observance, ventilation, and weather. In the end, he could find no differences between the clinics, other than the obvious fact that one was staffed by medical students and the other by midwifery students.

What were the midwives doing differently than the doctors? It turned out to be nothing, at least nothing related to how they cared for their patients on the maternity ward. The childbirth techniques were identical. It was what they did *on the way* to the ward that was different. The medical students spent their mornings doing autopsies; the midwives did not.

The clincher for Semmelweis came with the unfortunate death of one of his colleagues. This physician fell ill after being pricked by a scalpel—wielded by a medical student, no less—during an autopsy, and died shortly thereafter. Semmelweis participated in the autopsy of his colleague and noted that the pathology was identical to that of women dying from puerperal fever.

Although the germ theory of disease wasn't accepted yet and Semmelweis could not have known that it was streptococcal bacteria that were doing the dirty work, he concluded that "cadaveric particles" of some sort were being transferred on the medical students' hands from the autopsy room to the maternity ward. In May 1847, Semmelweis instructed his students to wash their hands with carbolic acid upon entry to the ward. The mortality rate in the First Clinic immediately plunged to that of the Second Clinic.

In the annals of medicine, this episode has gone down as one of the first successful patient-safety interventions. Semmelweis measured the problem, instituted a change, and measured the result. It had the potential to save untold numbers of lives. However, the Semmelweis tale is a cautionary one about implementation. You might have the best patient-safety intervention in the world—and arguably Semmelweis did—but if you don't implement it well, it's a lost cause.

Semmelweis faced resistance from the medical establishment, as anyone who disrupts the accepted order likely would. The senior Viennese doctors took umbrage that this Hungarian transplant—Jewish, no less—was insinuating that their esteemed medical care was actually *causing* the deaths of their patients. Shifting an accepted mind-set is a tall order, but it is a necessary one if you want to make any change. This requires finding the sweet spot between persuading, convincing, encouraging, and pressuring. Semmelweis evidently possessed none of these skills.

For starters, he didn't publish his findings for more than a decade, so no other doctors could examine his data. He insisted that they take his word for it, which irritated them even more. By all accounts, Semmelweis was abrasive and arrogant. He took critiques personally, responding to his colleagues' skepticism with public hectoring and insults. To one doctor, he wrote, "You, Herr Professor, have been a partner in this massacre."[15]

Beyond the personal acrimony there was the systems issue—if doctors had to wash their hands before examining patients, then there had to be sinks everywhere. The hospital plumbing systems would have to be completely reengineered, a hurdle that was not easily surmounted. Semmelweis finally published a book about puerperal fever some fifteen years after his initial experiment. His book was poorly received by a medical community still convinced that disease was caused by deleterious "miasmas" in the air. Ultimately the establishment derided and ignored Semmelweis and his ideas.

Semmelweis's mental condition thereafter rapidly deteriorated. It's not clear if he had Alzheimer's disease, bipolar disorder, or neurosyphilis, but there's no doubt that his condition was exacerbated by excessive stress (along with excessive alcohol). He spent the remaining four years of his life bitterly lashing out at the medical establishment, sending furious and insulting letters to his colleagues. He was committed to an insane asylum in 1865 and was dead within two weeks.

The supreme and painful irony was that although Semmelweis was ill when he arrived at the asylum, his death was almost surely hastened by the medical care he was given. When he tried to escape the asylum, he was severely beaten by guards, straightjacketed, and placed in isolation. Standard psychiatric treatments at the time included ice baths, purging, blistering, and bloodletting. By some accounts, the beating caused a wound on his hand that became infected and gangrenous in the poor conditions of the asylum.

Semmelweis likely died of sepsis, in the same manner as his patients in Vienna's First Clinic.

---

The Semmelweis affair is a case study in the critical importance of implementation when it comes to engineering patient safety. But there are other lessons to be learned from this, not least of which is to pay attention to what the nurses are doing. Just as the First Clinic was enjoying its first few years of lower mortality rates by emulating the midwives, a young Florence Nightingale was visiting hospitals throughout Europe and taking furious notes on their (mostly horrific) conditions. She noted that many medical treatments—which included arsenic, mercury, and the rampant bloodletting—inflicted more harm than good. Like Semmelweis, she quickly learned that doctors do not want to hear that their well-honed treatments are wrong, harmful, or both.

During the Crimean War, Nightingale worked in the British Army hospital in the Scutari region of the Ottoman Empire, and she was appalled by the abysmal conditions. At least four times as many soldiers died of disease as on the battlefield—numbers that came to light only because of Nightingale's meticulous record-keeping. She set rigorous standards for hygiene (including handwashing), wound care, food preparation, medical supplies, and patient triage. Over the course of 1855, the mortality rate in the hospital dropped sharply, from 33% to 2%.

In her 1863 book, *Notes on Hospitals*, she wrote with a rather modern style of pithy irony: "It may seem a strange principle to enunciate as the very first requirement in a hospital that it should do the sick no harm. It is quite necessary, nevertheless, to lay down such a principle." Nightingale's book preceded the IOM's *To Err Is Human* by 136 years, but the gist of the message was similar: medical care can actually be dangerous for patients and one must focus on fixing the system in order to improve overall health and safety. Nightingale was a bit more canny in her implementation approach than Semmelweis: she hand-delivered a copy of her book to Queen Victoria. As any modern-day patient-safety advocate can tell you, it always helps to go straight to the top brass.

There was pushback from the establishment, of course. Nightingale's experience was eerily similar to Peter Pronovost's a century and a half later with catheter-related infections: the medical profession had trouble accepting the idea that these bad outcomes were preventable. Just as it was accepted wisdom that catheter-related infections simply came with the territory, so were deaths in military hospitals considered part and parcel of war. Nightingale noted with angry resignation that the "sound principles of Hygiene are by no means widely spread" because people continued to accept "contagion as an unavoidable cause of death."[16] The idea that how we care for patients can cause harms was just as threatening to the medical establishment in the 1850s as it was in the early 2000s.

Nightingale also demonstrated—with just as much resistance—the same point that Pronovost had to argue, that you have to *measure* what's going on in order to know where, how, and if you can make progress. The military bureaucracy was apoplectic with frustration at Nightingale's insistence on detailed record-keeping, but she persevered. Many credit her with laying the foundations for modern-day infection control.

It's almost ironic that all five steps in Pronovost's checklist are present in Nightingale's own formula for improving patient care. He used the word "sterile" where she used the word "clean," but otherwise her rules are essentially the same—wash hands, clean the patient's skin, use clean coverings for the patient, use clean clothing for the staff, cover the wound with clean dressing.

From rigorous documentation and scrupulous clinical technique to a focus on systems improvement and implementation, it's no wonder Pronovost became so convinced of the need to empower nurses in order to tackle patient safety. Pronovost described to me how enlightened he'd considered himself at the beginning of his career. "I'll be a team player and I'll ask the nurses for their input" he'd told himself, congratulating himself on this progressive attitude. He sort of did, but it was really only lip service; he didn't actually listen to what they had to say. As he became more steeped in the culture of patient safety, he then decided to ask nurses to join doctors on rounds, because this would emphasize that medical care was a team effort. But the ICU was a busy place and it was often hard to coordinate. If the nurses weren't available at the time of rounds, it didn't make sense to delay everything, so he would go on without them.

"Now," he told me, "if the nurses aren't available, I won't do rounds at all."

Collaboration, he realized, wasn't just a politically correct buzzword, it was actually one of the most important pillars of patient safety. Staff members from different disciplines and different ranks needed to be able to work together and talk openly. They had to be able to point out problems and errors without fear of being reprimanded or belittled. If an institution is going to truly recognize the high-risk nature of medicine and commit to improving patient safety, it has to create an environment that fosters real collaboration. This requires a commitment of resources—you need to have adequate time, space, and staff. (Overstretched staff who can barely keep their heads above water won't have much bandwidth for collaboration.) It also requires a commitment of attitude—setting the example from the top that criticism is encouraged, that scapegoating won't be tolerated, that hierarchy and egos won't rule the day.

---

Patient safety and avoidance of medical error is a complex mix of how individual medical professionals interact and communicate with one another, how they do so with patients and family members, and how state-of-the-art medical systems can nevertheless allow small things to fall through the cracks. Human psychology plays as potent a role in the success (or failure) of medical care as the most advanced technologies. There's also a thread that carries forward from the stories of Semmelweis, Nightingale, and Pronovost: pay attention to the nurses. This is something that plays out potently in the story of Jay.

# CHAPTER TWO

# A SEA OF
# UNCERTAINTY

Not every naval aviator is game enough to give it a go at the Hula-Hoop, but Jay did not intimidate easily. Facing off against the Wii Fit Hula-Hoop game, there was the lieutenant commander in nothing but his boxers, gyrating his hips like a belly dancer in the family basement on a Friday morning in late May. As a naval reservist who flew in E-2C Hawkeye turboprops, Jay had to pass a grueling fitness test every six months, so he was always sniffing out creative ways to stay in shape. What could be better on a warm spring morning than Hula-Hooping in your skivvies?

A lean six-footer who didn't smoke, drink, or get sick, Jay was a relentless straight arrow. At thirty-nine, he was in as good physical shape as when he'd graduated from the Naval Academy. His day job was as a bank manager, and he dressed the part, even on weekends. But he had an easy laugh and an even easier smile.

The Hula-Hoop, though, is not for the faint of heart, especially without proper gear. On Saturday morning, Jay was feeling its effects. "My nuts are sore," he confided to his wife, Tara, confessing his boxer-shorts faux pas. She told him to call his doctor, but he shrugged it off. As an experienced ER nurse, Tara had handled many a weekend warrior with pulled groin muscles. She rattled off the basic treatment: jock strap, ice packs, ibuprofen (with food, please). And lay off the Hula-Hoop for a few days!

Tara had an ER shift the next day, and so she tiptoed out of the house while Jay and the kids were still sleeping. But around 9:30 on that Sunday morning, Jay called Tara and said his pain was now 8 out of 10 and he was nauseated. Tara told him to get to the hospital ASAP for an ultrasound because these could be signs of testicular torsion, a certifiable emergency. If a testicle is not surgically untwisted, it can die from lack of oxygen. This time, Jay complied.

In the emergency room, however, the ultrasound showed no torsion. A slew of routine labs clocked in as normal, with the exception of a slightly low white-blood-cell count. The pain was chalked up to overly exuberant exercise and the lieutenant commander was sent home with ibuprofen and ice packs.

White blood cells serve as the public face of the body's immune system. The various subtypes of white cells—neutrophils, lymphocytes, monocytes, basophils, eosinophils—each have specialized roles in protecting the body against bacteria, viruses, parasites, cancer, and allergens.

The white count—as it's usually referred to—is typically *elevated* when there is an infection. But some infections can lower the white count. When Jay's urine culture grew E. coli, urinary infection seemed a reasonable explanation. Jay was given ten days of ciprofloxacin, an antibiotic, with a plan to repeat the white count when the course of treatment was completed. After a day or two sitting on ice packs, Jay's groin pain resolved and he was back at work at the bank.

The repeat labs, though, showed an even lower white count. Within a few days Jay and Tara were sitting in a hematologist's office puzzling over the results. And it *was* a puzzle, as Dr. Selwin pointed out. Jay was squeaky-clean healthy. He had no fever, weight loss, or swollen lymph nodes. He had no rashes or joint pains. He hadn't traveled recently to an exotic locale or received a blood transfusion or gotten a tattoo from a seedy parlor or taken strange herbal remedies purchased off the Internet. He was just a little bit tired. And when you are raising two teenagers, working long hours in a bank, and keeping up as a naval reservist on the side, well, you'd be expected to be a little tired.

The clinical picture did not fit the profile of serious illnesses such as leukemia or HIV that can present with a very low white count. Statistically speaking, the low white-blood-cell count was most likely due to an ordinary viral syndrome. The other possibility was a condition called cyclic neutropenia, in which the white cells periodically drop, likely from a genetic disorder. In either case, the hematologist thought it would make sense to give Jay a dose of filgrastim, a bone marrow stimulant, just to get his white count out of the danger zone.

But this didn't feel right to Tara. Jay had always been perfectly healthy, and he didn't really have any symptoms of a viral syndrome. The urinary infection had been fully treated. Why should his white count be low? She asked Dr. Selwin to do a bone marrow biopsy to figure out what was going on inside. Dr. Selwin hesitated.

A bone marrow biopsy involves inserting an intimidatingly large needle into the hipbone to extract a sample of the marrow and inner bone. The bone marrow is the hive where the blood cells of the body develop, so a biopsy permits doctors to examine the immature forms of the blood cells. They can see if the cells appear aberrant (as they do in cancers such as leukemia and lymphoma). They can also see if the bone marrow has stopped producing blood cells altogether, which can occur as a result of infections, medications, toxins, radiation, genetic abnormalities, autoimmune disorders, or certain vitamin deficiencies.

So when it comes to figuring out why blood cells aren't behaving as they should, the bone marrow is where the money is. But it's not a minor procedure. When I was a resident at Bellevue Hospital at the height of the AIDS epidemic, our wards were filled to the gills with feverish patients who had abnormal blood counts and needed bone marrow biopsies, way more than the overworked hematology fellow could possibly keep up with. Waiting around for the fellow to be available drove me crazy. Besides delaying care for my patients, it delayed discharges, which kept my patient load high. So the only practical recourse, I decided, was to just learn to do it myself.

I tagged along with the kindly but exhausted hematology fellow for a week. There were so many bone marrow biopsies to do that I quickly got enough procedures under my belt to start doing them for my own patients. Of course, when word got out that I was certified in bone marrow biopsies, I was soon doing them for everyone's patients. I began stocking the biopsy kits in my locker (underneath my supply of granola bars) so that I wouldn't have to keep running down to central supply each time I needed one.

The thing that struck me most about the bone marrow biopsy was how physical a procedure it was. Most medical procedures I'd done to that point—spinal taps, arterial lines, central venous catheters, removing fluid from swollen abdomens or lungs—were delicate transactions that required a deft and careful touch. A bone marrow biopsy, on the other hand, required brute force.

A six-inch needle the width of a ballpoint pen is pressed through the patient's skin and soft tissue into the hipbone. Local anesthesia is used, of course, but the needle needs to be forced, corkscrew-like, deep into the bone. It's like twisting a wine-bottle opener into granite. You have to bear down and twist with real muscle to get that needle several centimeters into the hipbone. True, only the outer layer of bone—the periosteum—possesses nerve receptors and can detect pain, but the intense pressure of a doctor grinding deep into the bone is not lost on the patient. Or the doctor.

So I understood why Jay's hematologist didn't jump to a bone marrow biopsy willy-nilly. It's an invasive and painful procedure, with risks of infection and bleeding, so should be done only with careful thought. Dr. Selwin said he didn't think Jay needed one, or at least didn't need one yet. Jay didn't have any symptoms of a malignancy or severe infection (fever, weight loss, swollen lymph nodes). "Besides," Dr. Selwin pointed out, "what happens if I do the bone marrow biopsy and then it turns out not to be covered by your insurance? You could be stuck with a $5,000 bill."

Tara could see that Dr. Selwin was thinking about the whole patient, not just his narrow sliver of expertise, and she appreciated that. She'd seen him at work in the hospital—he was conscientious and thorough. But she just wasn't comfortable with the low white count. She pressed him to do the bone marrow biopsy.

Dr. Selwin's preference was to give the filgrastim a chance before deciding whether Jay truly needed a biopsy. But he'd also seen Tara's clinical instincts and her willingness to go the extra mile for his patients. "Okay," he finally said. "For you, I'll do it."

When the diagnosis came back as acute myeloid leukemia (AML), Dr. Selwin was as shocked as anyone. AML is a cancer of the white blood cells, and as its name suggests, it usually presents acutely. Patients with AML suffer raging fevers, drenching sweats, grinding fatigue, and bleeding gums. They can present in leukemic crisis in which floods of cancerous cells unleash hemorrhages, blood clots, overwhelming infections, respiratory distress, kidney failure, heart attacks, and strokes. Most patients newly diagnosed with AML are not capable of standing with crisp military posture, or piloting airplanes, or doing the Hula-Hoop. "I can't believe it myself," Dr. Selwin said.

---

The Brownian motion of life has a way of knocking seemingly irreconcilable events up against each other. And so it was that twenty-four hours after AML had macheted into their lives, Jay and Tara were seated amid a picturesque field of wildflowers, posing for a photographer with their two children. Tara had arranged this family portrait months earlier, because fifteen-year-old Sasha was setting off in two days for a once-in-lifetime trip to China. Sasha had been studying Mandarin in earnest, and she was now embarking on a month-long language-immersion program.

With raw and ragged emotions, Jay and Tara perched on a quaint stone bench, while Sasha and thirteen-year-old Chris goofed around behind them, mugging for the camera. Tara and Jay had made the difficult decision to not tell their children about the diagnosis just yet. They wanted Sasha to enjoy her long-planned trip with an unburdened heart. Jay and Tara gripped hands tightly during the photo shoot and leaned their heads together—his dark-brown hair against her red—while their children teased each other and cracked jokes. "We bolstered the weight of the world on our shoulders," Tara recalled, "to shield our children from this painful reality." The portrait shows a beautiful smiling family surrounded by a profusion of pink and purple flowers, with an old wooden fence sagging comfortably nearby.

Two days later they saw Sasha off at the airport. Holding their own emotions painfully in check, Tara and Jay hugged their daughter and sent her off on her long-anticipated adventure.

The hospital where Dr. Selwin and Tara worked did not have a specialized unit for leukemia, so Jay was referred to a big-city cancer center and that's where Jay and Tara found themselves shortly after they'd bid farewell to Sasha. For this initial consultation they were encouraged to bring family members, so the conference room was packed with Tara's and Jay's siblings, parents, and brothers- and sisters-in-law, all seated around a richly textured oak table.

Tall and good-natured, Dr. Everett took the time to get introduced to everyone in the sprawling family and genially tolerated everyone's eccentricities. But he was also blunt. He wanted to admit Jay to the hospital right away, as soon as the meeting ended, in fact, to begin chemotherapy.

Jay's robust health and lack of classic AML symptoms were good news, Dr. Everett said. The fact that Jay's labs—other than the low white count—were all normal was also good news. The fact that he hadn't experienced any infections or bleeding was more good news. All of these factors improved his odds. A true prognosis could not be entertained, of course, until the specific subtype of AML was known, but that wasn't any reason to delay the start of treatment.

AML is actually a conglomerate of subtypes, some that are known to be curable and others that carry graver prognoses. Although Jay's subtype wasn't known yet, an otherwise healthy person like him was the kind of patient for whom a cure was possible, even probable. Jay would ultimately require a bone marrow transplant, but doctors could fashion it from his own cells (an autologous transplant). They would harvest some of Jay's cells and protect them while the rest of his bone marrow was ablated by chemotherapy. When things settled down, they'd give Jay back his own cells to repopulate his bone marrow. There are always potential bumps along the way when it comes to removing, ablating, and restoring someone's immune system, but it was all eminently doable. Given the possibility of a full cure, chemotherapy should be started now. Today.

But there was a hitch. A uniquely American hitch. The kind of hitch that occurs only in places where the fine print of insurance policies can end up directing medical care. Jay had been at his current job for fifty-one weeks—a week shy of the one-year mark that he needed in order to qualify for short-term disability. If they started the chemotherapy now, he would be rendered ineligible for disability payments.

When Jay had first been told of the AML diagnosis by Dr. Selwin a week earlier, tears ran down his face. The first question he'd asked the doctor, in a quivering voice, was, "What will happen to my kids?"

And that question was still at the forefront of his mind. He and Tara knew that the treatment was not going to be easy—physically, mentally, or finan-cially. As it was, Jay and Tara were still recovering from Jay's job layoff a year earlier. They'd reluctantly uprooted their children from the only home they'd ever known and driven fifteen hours to relocate near a new job and grand-parents. At the time of the AML diagnosis, they were still living with Tara's parents, trying to save money to buy a house. Even with health insurance, a major illness could drain their savings.

And who knew what Jay would feel like at the end of his treatment and whether he'd be able to return to his job at the same level. Tara was putting in fifty to sixty-five hours per week in the ER, but even that might not be enough to support a family of four. Jay could be out of work for months, maybe even a year. Disability payments might be critical to their survival. The uncertainties of his health were agonizing enough. Jay didn't want to risk giving his family an additional hardship if there was a way to provide some sort of financial cushion. All on account of seven days . . .

So Jay asked his new hematologist if they could delay the start of treatment by one week. Dr. Everett hesitated. In the scheme of things, given the months and years it takes for a cancer to develop biologically, seven days probably wouldn't make a difference. But once you are in the ring, as it were, you never want to give cancer even the slightest edge.

But then again, you also don't want to pull the financial rug out from under a family about to embark on one of the most wrenching, frightening journeys imaginable. And how awful to put a patient in the horrific position of choosing between his health and his family's financial well-being. As a phy-sician, you want your patient to be in an emotionally strong position before embarking on a treatment course like this. Chemotherapy is a bulldozer, and it's not just the patient who feels the effects.

Luckily, all of Jay's good prognostic factors—young age, excellent health, lack of symptoms—were a buffer. The AML hadn't exploded yet, and there was no sign that this was imminent. Clinically, there wasn't any good reason that they couldn't wait seven days.

"This would be highly unusual," Dr. Everett said, but he agreed to post-pone the first treatment—induction chemotherapy—for a week.

"Game on!" Jay wrote on July 1 in the blog he'd begun keeping for his family and close friends. "Well, all we know right now is that it's AML, a type of Leukemia. I will be tested tomorrow (bone marrow again!) to determine if I have APML. This would be the best type of AML to have. The doctors don't think it's this one but I can keep my fingers crossed. Either way I will probably start my first round of Chemo next Wednesday."

July 1, coincidentally, is also *game on* for all the new interns, residents, and fellows in the hospital. It's the first day of the new medical year, so everyone is ratcheted up a notch on July 1. (I'll talk about the so-called "July effect"—if there actually is one—later on in the book.) The calendar coincidence did not go unnoticed by Tara. She was always vigilant as a nurse, but she was extra vigilant in July.

Jay called the benefits office at his job and verified that he would qualify for disability on July 8. The family health insurance was through Tara's job, so she would need to keep working in the ER during his treatment. While waiting for July 8 to arrive, Jay did the repeat bone marrow biopsy for the subtype testing. "Well it was a fun filled day today," Jay wrote in his blog. "They drilled into my hip again for bone marrow. We will get the tests back on Tuesday, but that is the fun part."

He also learned his tolerance—or lack thereof—for drugs. "I am truly a light-weight," he wrote. He'd been given some moderate-level pain medications before the procedure, and when it was all done, he promptly passed out in the elevator on his way home. After some fluids and monitoring, he was sent on his way. He quipped on his blog that he'd make a lousy drug dealer.

Induction chemotherapy is the most powerful round of chemotherapy, intended to obliterate the cancerous cells as forcefully and definitively as possible. Despite all of our medical advances, however, chemotherapy is still a crude instrument. It drops like an anvil on rapidly dividing cells—the sine qua non of cancerous cells—but in its wake will mow down all other rapidly dividing cells in the body, such as bone marrow cells, hair cells, and the cells that line the mouth, stomach, and entire gastrointestinal tract. Hence the cardinal side effects of chemotherapy—nausea, vomiting, mouth ulcers, hair loss, plus decimation of red blood cells, platelets, and healthy white cells. Loss of these cells leads to anemia, bleeding, and infections.

As such, induction chemotherapy is usually done as inpatient treatment so that the patient can be monitored closely for these potentially deadly side effects. (Subsequent rounds of chemotherapy with milder doses can often be done on an outpatient basis.)

Jay and Tara waited nervously through that first week in July but endeavored to keep the home routine normal. They sat down with thirteen-year-old Chris and told him about Jay's diagnosis. They explained that Daddy would be very sick for the next few weeks but that he would be getting good medical care from his doctors and nurses. They explained that they would tell Sasha about it when she got home from her trip in China. They kept things as calm and low-key as possible. As it happened, Chris had a weeklong sleep-away camp coming up. Jay and Tara agreed that it would be good for him to be with his friends and not to have to witness the harsh first round of chemotherapy. They helped him pack and kept up their smiles as they saw him off on the bus.

The day before Jay's admission to the hospital for induction chemo, the extended family gathered to help him shave his head. Tara's five siblings, plus spouses and parents, assembled under the majestic maple tree in her parents' front yard. It was lighthearted and wrenching all at the same time. Tara's father sang in Italian like a barber as he tried to give Jay a buzz cut. The clippers jammed in the middle of his aria, and they had to dig out regular scissors. The crew of barbers was ridiculously inexperienced and the process took more than an hour. Jay—who'd been through the head-shaving routine multiple times in the military—tolerated his motley groomers good-naturedly. Between the goofiness and jokes, though, each family member was overcome with tears at some point and quietly excused him- or herself to weep in a distant part of the yard.

Tara's sister snapped a photo of Jay just before the shaving ceremony began. Jay's eyes crinkle at the corners and he almost looks mischievous. There was no fear apparent in his two-hundred-watt smile. But hours later, at one in the morning, he rolled his face into Tara's chest, sobbing. "I'm scared," he told her. His body was shaking, and all Tara could do was reassure him that he wouldn't be alone. She caressed the smooth skin of his head, holding her own fears inside so as not to worsen his anxiety. Jay finally drifted off, while Tara remained awake trying to wrestle away her fears.

The next morning, July 8, Tara and Jay drove an hour to the cancer center for the induction chemotherapy. "This place will become my second home for the next two years," Tara remembered thinking. For a facility with such a high reputation, it was shabbier than she'd expected. The ceiling tiles were stained, the walls dented, and the flooring reminiscent of the 1950s. But Tara had worked in enough hospitals to know that externalities ultimately had no bearing on quality. She'd worked with fantastic medical staff in the unfanciest of settings. Coming in as a patient, though, made you see things a little differently. A little window dressing wouldn't have hurt.

"The Games Begin!" Jay had written in his blog the night before. And begin they did. Jay was whisked straight to the interventional radiology suite to get an indwelling catheter implanted in his chest. This would stay semi-permanently for the duration of his chemotherapy, minimizing the need for dozens of needle-sticks and IVs. Tara watched with relief when Jay was wheeled back on a stretcher, deep in conversation with the burly orderly, asking the orderly how many children he had and how old they were.

The site of the catheter placement was sore, and the pain worsened over the course of the afternoon. "They gave me some pain meds," Jay wrote later that day, "and guess who passed out again! Now the most they'll give me is Tylenol!"

Once the catheter was placed, Jay was ready to start his chemo. But when Dr. Everett arrived, there was bad news. The final results of Jay's bone marrow biopsy showed a mutation known as trisomy 11—a rarer and nastier form of AML. Dr. Everett, who had seemed so jovial and upbeat at their initial meeting, was all business now as he related this grimmer news. Chemotherapy would still start today, but he would rejigger the components to take this new information into account. And Jay would not be able to use his own bone marrow for a transplant—they'd need to turn to the family for donors.

The week of the induction chemotherapy was brutal. All the textbook side effects showed up like clockwork—nausea, vomiting, mouth sores, plummeting blood counts. Tara ran back and forth between Jay's hospital and hers, keeping up as many ER shifts as she could. Her five siblings and their spouses and their in-laws tag-teamed with Jay's work colleagues and Tara's parents so that Jay was never alone during this rough week.

"Thank you for the inspirational notes and the visits," Jay wrote in the blog. "It's nice to have people come and go and just watch a movie. Plus in my new condition I ask much more personal questions, since what do I have to lose? I have cancer—you have to answer me now! :-) "

The thing Jay feared most was being helpless. He was determined not to turn into one of those hollow-eyed patients he'd seen in movies, who could barely muster the energy to sip ginger ale through a bendy straw. So no matter how rotten he felt, every few hours he lugged his IV pole and made his rounds of the floor. Tara joked that it was like he was running for office, the way he greeted each and every person he passed, each and every time.

"Feeling pretty good right now," Jay wrote, several days into the chemo. "Think I have the right mix of nausea and chemo drugs going on. Tara and I are about to start my evening walk. Going to do about 1/4 mile."

Jay was on the BMTU—the bone marrow transplant unit—even though he wasn't yet getting a bone marrow transplant. The BMTU was the central location for all hematology patients with leukemia. Dr. Chowdury, the heme-onc fellow, was in charge of Jay's day-to-day care in the BMTU. Tara recalled that Dr. Chowdury spent more quality time in Jay's room than anyone else, even more time than the nurses (high praise, indeed, coming from a nurse). For Jay and Tara, Dr. Chowdury's presence was instantly calming and reassuring. Her unhurried style, her willingness to answer every question, and her genuine caring were a lifeline during those stressful days. Dr. Everett was the attending guiding Jay's overall treatment but Dr. Chowdury was the boots-on-the-ground doc who was on the BMTU all day, every day.

"I hope you are all doing as well as I am, LOL," Jay wrote, midway through the chemo. "My chin is up. The tough days will be coming and I am ready for the fun. Lips won't be good and neither will the end where the sun don't shine. But I know I can handle it. . . ."

Two days later, Jay wrote, "Well, I must really be settling into a schedule now. I woke up at 5:30, shaved, then went for my 13-lap walk along with some Wii Fit exercises. It feels good to tire my legs and abs a bit. Makes me feel alive.

"Feeling good, but not tasting so good. The chemo taste in my mouth is a bit much right now. But I will trade bad taste any day I can exercise."

On July 13, on last day of chemo, Tara arrived in the evening after her shift. It had been a long day, and she soon fell asleep on the couch in Jay's room. She awoke at 3 a.m. and her eyes, per usual, went right to Jay. She sprang off the couch when she realized that Jay's bed was empty. She found him in the bathroom, struggling to untwist his tangled IV lines. As she reached to help with the IVs she noticed a strange look on his face. His skin was pale and sweaty, and before she could even say anything, he began to have a seizure. Tara caught his body as he collapsed, but they both tumbled to the floor. Every hospital bathroom has a call button, but Tara—pinned beneath her six-foot husband—couldn't reach it. She screamed for help, but the bathroom door was closed, and Jay's room was more than thirty yards from the nurses' station.

Tara struggled to extricate herself from her husband's shuddering body, shimmying and crawling until she could just reach the call button. A nurse came quickly, and her immediate calls for help brought in a posse of other nurses plus the overnight heme-onc fellow, Dr. Amir.

Tara recalled being surprised that nobody wheeled in a code cart or oxygen, but they did perform an EKG, which showed a very low heart rate—thirty beats per minute. The working explanation was that the slow heart rate caused syncope (fainting), which in turned caused the seizure.

The next day both a cardiologist and a neurologist came to see Jay. A CT scan of the head and a tilt-table test (to evaluate causes of fainting) were negative and both doctors "cleared" Jay. Dr. Everett was away, but the covering hematologist was in agreement that all of this was a side effect of chemo, and the next day Jay was discharged home.

Tara argued that should this happen again at home, Jay could easily fall and smash his head. She thought Jay should stay at least another day in the hospital. But the covering hematologist felt that the risk of infection should Jay stay longer in the hospital far outweighed the risk of falling.

The first days at home were relatively uneventful. Jay had an armada of anti-everything to take—anti-fungals, anti-virals, anti-emetics, antacids, and, of course, antibiotics. Now that the chemotherapy had rolled, tank-like, over his immune system, he was a sitting duck for infection. Home was less dangerous than the hospital in this regard, but it was still a risk. Every hiccup, every dust mite, every smudge could harbor a potentially deadly pathogen. The medications were an attempt to weave a web of protection, but no web is ever solid. Jay and Tara had to check his temperature round the clock, remaining vigilant for even the slightest fever, with instructions to return to the hospital immediately when the thermometer hit 100.4 degrees. "It's not a matter of *if*," said his doctor, "but *when* you get a fever."

"Up again in the middle of the night," Jay wrote at 4:00 a.m. on his second night at home. "Don't feel bad for me, as I am still at home which is awesome. More choices on TV and the Internet is better! I am really feeling weak due to my low blood counts and had to pass on a shower today. Tara was nice enough to get me cleaned up. Wow, a great wife and a nurse! I highly recommend sponge baths, but not if you need to get leukemia to get one . . ."

Two days later, Jay was feeling stronger, so Tara helped him take a much-needed and much-desired shower. They were easing into the shower stall when suddenly Jay began to wobble and his eyes rolled back in his head. Tara braced herself to catch him as he started to lose consciousness. He landed with a thud against her. She was able to guide him down to the floor slowly but was once again pinned beneath him. She yelled for her mother to come help, but when she turned her head, she saw that it was their son standing in doorway. Tara forced her voice to calm down. "It's all okay, Chris. Daddy's okay, but I just need Grandma's help now. Please get her now." When Tara's mother arrived in the bathroom, they laid Jay flat and elevated his legs. Jay regained consciousness quickly and was devastated that his son had to witness this. His first words were, "Please go take care of Chris."

That night, Chris parked himself near the couch where his father slept. He set out his sleeping bag just a few inches from where Tara was bedding down on the floor and spent the night there. Tara was heartbroken to see how much the episode in the shower had rattled her son.

It rattled her too. This was now Jay's third episode of syncope. Tara was less concerned about the *cause* of the loss of consciousness—he'd already had a full evaluation from a cardiologist and neurologist in the hospital—than that it could happen at a random time. What if she hadn't been right next to him in the shower? If he slammed his head on a wall or on the floor going down, he could easily hemorrhage into his brain. With his platelet counts decimated by the chemo, the bleeding could be unstoppable.

Tara had helped so many patients and families deal with illness, but this was the first time she herself had descended into the existential panic that comes with serious disease. There was nothing that could offer a bedrock of certainty—not her nursing experience, not the hematology textbook she'd checked out of the medical library, not the skills or qualifications of Jay's doctors—nothing. The terrifying truth is that when you or a family member gets sick—no matter how many friends and family are there for you, no matter how superb the medical team is—you are still alone in a sea of uncertainty.

CHAPTER THREE

# MAKING — OR MISSING — THE DIAGNOSIS

I t was another one of those bursting-at-the-seams types of days in my clinic. Every scheduled patient showed up, plus a few extra added on. Everybody seemed to have burning concerns that needed immediate attention. One patient had newly diagnosed thyroid disease but the medication was making her feel worse rather than better. Another was having strange twinges in his lower abdomen. One woman had muscle aches in her arms that were now extending to her legs. Another patient was experiencing drilling-type pain in his lower back that spread up to his neck and scalp. One man had a cough that just wouldn't leave. A woman was concerned because the soles of her feet felt like they were on fire. Another patient said that she simply had no energy and could hardly get through her day.

For each of these presenting symptoms there is a gamut of possible causes— what doctors call the "differential diagnosis"—that range from the prosaically benign to the concerningly urgent to the immediately life-threatening. The name of the game is to come up with a broad differential for each symptom, then prioritize them by likelihood and by severity. Testing for every possible diagnosis is not feasible, so the doctor needs to ask the right questions, listen carefully to the answers, do the right kind of physical exam, and pay attention to the clinical clues.

If you had the luxury of an hour with each patient, you would have the time to diligently sort through each and every possibility. But the reality is that you have just a few minutes to push the majority of diagnoses to the bottom of the list, come up with the most likely few at the top—being careful, of course, to keep in the rare but life-threatening possibilities—and then explain to the patient what you think. You can order labs, X-rays, and the like, but those results won't come until later. You need to offer the patient, right now, the most likely diagnoses, as well as a plan for how to start treatment and/or further investigation.

It's a tall order, and an incredibly stressful one. Most textbooks treat diagnosis as a leisurely intellectual process. Medical students are taught to run through each organ system of the body and then consider all the plausible ways that organ system can get pillaged—via trauma, via infection, via metabolic derangement, via cancerous transformation, via toxic exposure, via genetic abnormalities. It's a thrilling academic exercise, especially if pondered over with a steaming cup of tea and plate of crumpets with jam while the sun eases its languid way across the firmament. Gentle strains of Chopin in the background don't hurt either.

Unfortunately that is not the way differential diagnosis happens in real life. At best we have a minute or two to navigate the wide chasm of possibilities. For each patient, the presenting symptom could be nothing or could be something. Or could be something horrible. Was the patient with no energy just not getting enough sleep? Or was she anemic, or hypothyroid, or depressed? Could she be suffering from pancreatic cancer? Maybe she was experiencing domestic violence?

Was the patient with muscle aches experiencing a medication side effect or exhibiting the onset of a systemic inflammatory disease? Did the gentleman with abdominal twinges have vascular compromise to his intestines or was he a hypochondriac? Or was he taking some Slavic weight loss concoction he'd purchased on the Internet?

As I raced through my day, I struggled to be thorough while trying to avoid falling too woefully behind schedule. The ulcer gnawing at the pit of every doctor's stomach is "What if I miss something serious?"

General practitioners such as internists, family doctors, pediatricians, and emergency doctors face the biggest challenges because the diagnostic field is so wide open. We all want to get it right, but we also don't want to over-order tests that can be harmful or expensive or yield too many false positives or all of the above. We may want to allow some observation time to see if the symptoms self-resolve or progress, but then we worry about missing a serious illness, harming a patient, or getting sued. Some days it feels shocking that we get it right at all.

And we do, on average, get it mostly right. Doctors' diagnostic accuracy is estimated to be in the range of 90%.[1] That, of course, implies a 10% error rate, but on days when it feels like you are being pelted with diagnostic possibilities from every cell of the body and that imminent death is lurking everywhere you turn and you have only minutes to make those decisions, that 90% number is comforting.

On cooler-headed days, though, that 10% error rate is disturbing.

———

Thirteen years into my clinical practice as a doctor, I took a year-long writing sabbatical. While I was away, a new faculty member took over my patients. When I returned, I sat down with my colleague and got the notable updates on my patients. By all accounts, everything went smoothly during my year away. Then she paused. "There was one thing, though . . . " And from the tone of her voice I could tell it wasn't something good.

Ms. Romero was a 69-year-old woman who had been in my practice for several years. She was generally well, and our visits were mainly focused on helping her lose weight, exercising her arthritic joints, and adjusting her thyroid and blood pressure medications. Her adult daughter in her home country had suffered a devastating illness, and the stress of that dominated many of our visits.

"There was an anemia," my colleague said slowly. "And it looked like it was never worked up." Anemia? Not worked up? I could feel my gut starting to winch painfully. Had I missed an anemia? I fervently hoped it would turn out to be the mild-annoyance type of anemia, as most anemias are.

I was wrong.

"It turned out to be multiple myeloma," she informed me quietly, and my gut bottomed out to my ankles. I'd missed a cancer.

———

The differential diagnosis of anemia is as prodigious as it is varied. Anemia can be caused by deficiencies of nutrients such as iron, B12, or folate. It can be caused by heavy menses, or a bleeding stomach ulcer, or bleeding from anywhere. It can be caused by liver disease and kidney disease. It can also be caused by inflammatory disease, bone marrow disease, and, of course, by cancer. Red blood cells can rupture—hemolyze—and cause anemia. Alcohol, medications, and toxins can cause anemia. HIV and parvovirus B19 can cause anemia. Anemia can be a fellow traveler with a host of chronic diseases. The list is endless.

Ms. Romero didn't have any symptoms that might suggest some of the more obvious causes. Her other blood tests were basically normal, which ruled out a slew of other causes. She was up to date with her regular cancer-screening tests such as mammogram and colonoscopy, so it wasn't any of the obvious cancers.

Multiple myeloma is a blood cell cancer that normally trundles along in a protracted, indolent phase before it "presents." Patients typically come to medical attention because of bone pain and unexplained fractures. The other way it is often diagnosed is when a high calcium level is noted incidentally on a blood test for other reasons.

Ms. Romero never had any of these symptoms—she always felt fine when I saw her—and her calcium was always normal. But it was clear, in retrospect, that she had been quietly developing multiple myeloma during the years that she was under my care.

The family was very upset. Even though the treatment and prognosis weren't affected by the delay in diagnosis—given the slow biology of the disease—it was still devastating to them. They were angered that this hadn't been diagnosed earlier.

"I'm sorry to have to give you the bad news," my colleague said, not unkindly. "But if it were me, I'd want to know."

It hardly gets more horrible than missing a cancer. Beyond that, I felt I had violated my patient's trust in the most fundamental way. Ms. Romero had entrusted her health to me for all of these years, assuming that if she came regularly to her appointments I would make sure she would be okay.

Over the years I've written a lot about the power of emotions over intellect, but I'd never felt it as acutely as at that moment. The intellectual side of me wanted to immediately tear through Ms. Romero's chart with a fine-toothed comb to figure out exactly where and how I'd blundered. While I knew this couldn't change the outcome or undo the mistake, I needed to pinpoint my error. When I was doing my PhD in a biochemistry laboratory, every failed experiment was followed by a rigorous autopsy; it was the only way to do better in the future and it was simply the right thing to do.

And yet. . . .

And yet, I could not bring myself to do it now. My horror at missing this diagnosis, at letting down my patient (not to mention the shame of an error revealed publicly in all its glory) got the better of me. The emotions were so overpowering that I could not manage more than a cursory glance at Ms. Romero's chart.

Over the years that ensued, I occasionally caught sight of Ms. Romero in the clinic. (It was clear—and frankly appropriate—that she preferred to stay with my colleague rather than return to my practice as all my other patients had after I'd returned from my sabbatical.) Each time I spotted her, I so wanted to approach her—to apologize, to explain, even just to wish her well during this difficult journey. But I was torn. Would I be doing this for her or for me? Was I trying to make amends with honesty or was I just desperate to clear my own conscience?

I tried to imagine it from her perspective: Would my appearance, with however earnest an apology, be welcome or would it be an intrusion? Would I be offering balm for a festering wound or churning up old emotions that had already settled?

I knew from my own research into medical error that what patients typically most want is honest acknowledgment and apology from their doctors. But if Ms. Romero had already made peace over the years with her cancer and its diagnosis, my reappearance might serve only to unsettle the homeostasis. Would it actually help *her*, or was I being selfish, hoping she'd offer some sort of absolution to assuage *my* terrible guilt? And if my visit wasn't well received, I wouldn't be able to undo it.

It was that latter realization that made me decide not to approach her. I couldn't countenance the chance of harming her even more. Though maybe I was just making excuses to hide the fact that I was basically chickening out, unable to face my own incompetence straight on.

It was another five full years before I could bring myself to examine her chart in detail. I had just learned that Ms. Romero died—by all accounts peacefully, comfortably, at home with her family. I was heartsick about the whole situation, especially that I might have caused extra pain for Ms. Romero and her family, beyond even the misery of cancer itself.

Now it was time, I decided. I needed to face up to my error, even if belatedly and even if the error hadn't necessarily changed the outcome of the disease. It was still an error. I'd missed an anemia.

I pored over the chart obsessively, determined to do the analysis I'd been unable to attempt previously. I went at it voraciously, charting her clinical course almost to the day, vowing not to rest until I'd cornered my error and figured out how not to do it again.

In medicine, though, nothing is ever as clear as the textbooks. Diseases—and patients—never seem to follow those flow charts so confidently constructed in the canon of medicine.

---

Anemia is diagnosed by the hematocrit, which represents the percentage of the blood occupied by red blood cells, and has a fairly wide range of what is considered normal. Depending on the laboratory, normal can range from 39 to 50 for men and 36 to 46 for women, though many women live comfortably in the low-to-mid 30s due to continuing menstrual blood loss.

The hematocrit is measured as part of a CBC (complete blood count), which also includes the platelets that are involved in blood clotting and the white blood cells that are part of the body's immune system.

Despite the common practice of ordering "executive profiles"—broad arrays of lab tests that are done to "check everything"—there is, in fact, no reason for a CBC to be ordered for an asymptomatic adult patient. There is no clinical guideline that recommends routine CBCs because the risk of false positive values (abnormal results when in fact there is no disease) is so high. A CBC should be ordered only when there is a clinical reason to do so, such as a bleeding issue (to see if the hematocrit has dropped and to check for sufficient platelets for clotting), an infection (to check for an abnormal white count), or a new symptom of fatigue (to look for anemia). This stands in contrast to tests for things such as cholesterol, where there are particular age recommendations for routine screening and robust clinical data to back up the utility in asymptomatic patients.

There wasn't any reason for me to have ordered a CBC based on Ms. Romero's other conditions, so the few CBCs that were in her chart before I left for sabbatical were likely ordered by other people for other reasons (if she had come to the ER, for example, with a pneumonia).

There were one or two CBCs in the computer from nearly a decade earlier, and her hematocrit had been 37 or 38. Then, about five years before I left, she was admitted to the hospital for abdominal pain. At that time, a CBC was done—likely looking for an elevated white count that might suggest an infection. The hematocrit was 35 and the next day it was 31. An acute drop like that can be from active bleeding—but there was no evidence of that in the chart. In a hospital setting a drop in the hematocrit can also be an artificial drop after aggressive IV hydration. (Because the hematocrit is a percentage, it can appear to drop if you suddenly pump in a lot of fluid. The number of red blood cells—what you are actually concerned about—is still the same.)

The abdominal pain turned out to be nothing serious and Ms. Romero was discharged. For some reason, she did not get an appointment with me and was seen in the walk-in clinic the following month. The CBC was repeated, and now the hematocrit was back up to 35, basically the same as when she had been admitted to the hospital. That doctor may have attributed the drop to 31 to hydration, and now it was back to baseline. It was likely assumed she "lived" in the 35 range and that the 31 was a spurious value.

I can't say for sure, though, because the doctor's thought process was not documented in the chart. At my next visit with Ms. Romero I'd probably seen the results in passing and may have made the same assumption. But I can't confirm that, because I, too, hadn't written anything in my note from that day about the hematocrit. I probably hadn't seen any need to write out my thoughts on a presumably normal lab value.

Separate from the issue of how we doctors mentally viewed Ms. Romero's lab results, there's also the physical manner in which we viewed those results. In our EMR at that time, the first result in the set would come up, and the rest would plug through—one by one—as you hit the return key. In this manner you'd see the CBC, then the metabolic profile, then the liver function tests, then the thyroid test, etc. However, for each individual lab test, you could also select a Trend function, in which you could compare this lab test to similar ones in the past.

Trending is extremely helpful, for example, in following the blood sugars in someone who is diabetic, allowing you to observe the trend over time. But if a test is normal, there generally isn't a reason to take the extra steps to examine the trend. Even in EMRs that automatically compare current results to prior results, the default setting is usually just to the past few rounds of blood tests. To do the trend over a long period of time, you have to make a conscious decision.

When I did the trend on Ms. Romero's CBC now, I could see a gradual drift downward over the decade, but it obviously hadn't caught my eye in real time. Perhaps I'd only compared her CBC to the one just prior, and I'd never done the trend all the way back. Maybe I hadn't noticed the drift because I wasn't actively "following" her blood count over the years, as I might have been, say, for a woman with large uterine fibroids who was experiencing bleeding.

I could see in the chart that shortly before I left for my sabbatical, Ms. Romero had gone to the walk-in clinic for symptoms of dizziness. A CBC at that time showed a hematocrit of 30. The doctor who'd evaluated her noted that this was below her baseline of 35. But her dizziness resolved at a follow-up visit—it was attributed to a concomitant viral syndrome—and the hematocrit of 30 must have fallen off that doctor's radar.

When Ms. Romero saw me a few weeks later, the focus of the visit was on her ill daughter. In my note from that day, I had commented about the resolution of her dizziness. But there was nothing written about the hematocrit of 30. Perhaps I simply hadn't seen the CBC. Or maybe I had, but didn't do a trend to compare to the earlier values (though 30 is low enough that it should have caught my attention by itself). Or maybe she'd been weeping in my office about her daughter—as had happened before, and we'd spent the entire time processing her grief. Or maybe I was rushing and hadn't been as thorough as I should have been. I can't say.

Reconstructing my thinking about why one particular strand of hay did or did not stand out in my mind compared to all the other strands of hay in the vast haystack is impossible, especially for a medical encounter years ago amid hundreds, even thousands, of other medical visits I'd done. (Though this is precisely what is expected in malpractice cases.) I wished fervently that I could reconstruct my mind-set, but it would be intellectually dishonest to even intimate that I could. In reality, I have no idea what I thought at the time.

When my colleague took over Ms. Romero's case a few months later, she was seeing a "new" patient and so evaluated everything from scratch. The low hematocrit of 30 jumped out at her immediately and she repeated the test. It was now 23. The hematocrit had plummeted in the few months' gap of our handover of care, and it was now eminently clear that something was very wrong. At that point, the hematologists did additional testing, including a bone marrow biopsy, and rapidly made a diagnosis of multiple myeloma.

---

Ms. Romero's case has haunted me over the years. For doctors and nurses, it's devastating to have missed a serious diagnosis, and agonizing to contemplate the additional distress you've caused your patient, above and beyond the illness itself. I wish I could rewind my brain those many years to figure out how I missed it. Had I been distracted? Was I running behind? Was I cutting corners to catch up? Was I willfully ignoring the lab data? Was I just having a bad day?

I discussed the case with Hardeep Singh, an internist from Houston who heads up the patient-safety initiatives at the VA hospital there and is an internationally known guru on medical error. Singh pointed out that diagnostic error is a completely different can of worms from procedural error (e.g., surgery on the wrong side of the body or an infection from a central line) because diagnosis is a moving target. He defines diagnostic error as "a missed opportunity to make a correct or timely diagnosis," even if the patient isn't harmed by the delay. The question is whether you could have done something different.

"Diagnoses evolve over time," Singh explained. They also evolve over place and people, as patients sometimes see different doctors or go to different hospitals to continue their care. Autopsies, which used to be the way that the medical system unlocked the answers, have steeply declined because of financial priorities as well as cultural norms. This is partly why diagnostic accuracy is fiendishly difficult to measure precisely. "Doctors often have no way of knowing if they've made a diagnostic error or not," Singh said.

Take the case of abdominal pain. This symptom is a daily occurrence for clinicians who work in general medicine, emergency departments, or urgent-care centers. There are days when the presence of abdominal pain seems as ubiquitous as oxygen, and this ubiquity can sometimes dull the sense of urgency. But the differential diagnosis of abdominal pain is as extensive as it is varied. It ranges from the common (acid reflux) to the rare (porphyria), and from the benign (constipation) to the life-threatening (intestinal rupture).

When I talk with a patient and examine her abdomen, my mind runs through this list, prioritizing which diagnoses seem more likely but still trying to keep in mind the more serious conditions that I can't afford to miss, even if they are rare. Each additional thing the patient says—no blood in her stool, occasional nausea but no vomiting, no weight loss or fever—rejiggers the list in my head. Her background medical history—absence of cancer, presence of hypertension—as well as the medications she does or does not take, all enter the mix, causing the diagnoses to reshuffle yet again.

There are some situations in which getting the *exact* right answer isn't necessary. Just corralling the differential diagnosis into categories of serious versus non-serious is often sufficient, at least initially. If I can separate out those patients who don't have any "red flag signs," I can hold off on expensive tests and simply observe to see what happens. Many patients will get better with just the tincture of time, and for those who don't, I can then consider doing additional tests.

In other cases, it can be reasonable to proceed with a treatment even without a specific diagnosis. An acid blocker, for example, can treat both acid reflux and gastritis, so it often isn't necessary to do the tests to distinguish between them. Not making a specific diagnosis in this case would not be considered an error.

However, I often never learn the outcome because many patients don't come back. If they are feeling better, why bother? If they are feeling worse, they may head to an emergency room, or to another doctor. If that next doctor does an endoscopy and discovers a gastric ulcer containing the bacteria *H. pylori* (which would require antibiotics in addition to acid blockers), then I clearly made an error, right?

Not necessarily, according to Singh. It would depend on whether there had been a clue that I'd missed that should have directed me to order an endoscopy right away—if the patient was feeling full more quickly than usual, for example, or was losing weight or noticed blood in her stool. But there are many cases in which the symptoms are not concerning enough to warrant an invasive test initially, and observation is appropriate. If the symptoms don't improve, then at the next visit, the endoscopy is warranted. That an ulcer was found at that time wouldn't necessarily mean that I'd made a mistake initially. It simply illustrates that diagnoses are moving targets and often require a period of time before they can be pinned down. Doing an endoscopy on every single patient who comes to an internist with abdominal pain would certainly catch all those ulcers up front, but it would be a logistical—and financial—impossibility, given that nearly all human beings have abdominal pain at some point in their lives.

Moreover, endoscopies have side effects. The actual risk of major adverse events from endoscopy (infection, bleeding, tearing of the stomach or esophagus, cardiac arrest from the sedation) is low, something in the range of one in a thousand. But if you do endoscopies on the millions of people out there with abdominal pain, these devastating outcomes will start to add up. And if those endoscopies ultimately weren't necessary for the vast majority of patients, then you've simply exposed patients to harm without offering much benefit. That is why, in the absence of red flag signs, most doctors typically observe first and then consider endoscopies only if patients don't get better with basic treatment.

Much of medical error research focuses on the inpatient setting, when patients are hospitalized. Errors in the inpatient setting are often more dramatic and thus more easily come to light. There's also the convenience factor for researchers—patients and their medical teams are all tethered to one central location. Plus, there's a trove of data to work with, since inpatients endure boatloads of tests in concentrated time periods. The majority of medical care, however, takes place in the outpatient setting—in doctors' offices, clinics, and community health centers. In these settings it's far harder to identify diagnostic errors because patients may spend only fifteen minutes in the medical setting and then waltz off into their own lives, far from the clutches of researchers and their clipboards.

Slowly, though, the field is turning its lens to this more unwieldy side of medicine. Singh and his colleagues undertook a study to get a sense of the scope of diagnostic error in outpatient, primary care medicine. They quickly learned that it's much more challenging to track down errors when patients are free to go wherever they please, whenever they please. How would the researchers even know where to look for the errors? Nobody checks off "error" in the chart when there's a mistake.

Singh and his colleagues reasoned that patients who experience a misdiagnosis are probably more likely to need additional medical care soon, since their problem wasn't correctly identified at the outset.[2] They thus hypothesized that anyone getting a second round of medical care within two weeks of a first visit would be more likely to have experienced a diagnostic error.

The handy part about using this metric was that the researchers could create an automatic trigger in the EMR. For any visit to the doctor, a red flag would automatically go up if—within two weeks—that patient returned for more medical care, such as another doctor's visit, admission to the hospital, or a visit to the ER or urgent care. Obviously, it was of no help if the patient sought care in another system, but many patients stay within their system for insurance reasons or for simplicity of care.

For every case brought to light by the trigger, researchers would then delve manually into the chart to see if there was anything that pointed to diagnostic error in the first visit, or whether it was just happenstance that there were two medical evaluations within two weeks of each other. Out of 212,165 visits, the trigger uncovered 674 patients who were hospitalized and 669 patients who returned for another outpatient visit (to a doctor, urgent care, or an ER) within two weeks of their initial visit. The researchers compared these to 614 "control" visits that were not followed by additional medical care within two weeks.

The researchers took into account that many diagnoses evolve over time (e.g., symptoms that initially suggested a viral syndrome but after a week progressed to a pneumonia). These they did not consider errors. They looked for cases in which there was some clue in the initial visit that might have been overlooked (e.g., symptoms suggested a viral syndrome, but there was an abnormality on the lung exam). They categorized an error only when there was a missed opportunity to make an earlier diagnosis.

In the group of patients who ended up admitted to the hospital within two weeks of a visit, 21% had evidence of a diagnostic error. In the group that went to the ER, urgent care, or back to the doctor within two weeks, 5% had a diagnostic error. By comparison, only 2% of the control group had an error.

The most commonly missed diagnoses were pneumonia, heart failure, renal failure, cancer, and urinary infection. I was most taken with the observation that nearly all the errors (more than 80%) were related to a problem in the doctor-patient interaction (as opposed to errors related to tests or referrals or patient actions). This means that the problems—and the potential solutions—are grounded in how doctors and patients interact.

Singh and colleagues teased apart this interaction and found that the three elements that contributed the most to errors were the history, the physical, and the ordering of diagnostic tests. (Failure to fully review the patient's chart—which might have been my error with Ms. Romero—contributed, but to a lesser degree.) Although the history, the physical, and the ordering of tests feel like separate elements, they are really part and parcel of the unified thinking process that goes into evaluating a patient. It reinforces the idea that diagnostic error relates to *cognitive* errors—how we think. And of course, how we think is much less amenable to the checklist approach we can use in other areas of medical error.

The researchers noted that 80% of visits lacked a differential diagnosis. That is, in only one out of five visits did the doctor deliberatively consider alternative diagnoses in strong enough terms to document them in the chart.

Mark Graber, another leading researcher in the area of diagnostic error, sees this statistic as the core of the problem. "Doctors need the discipline of the differential diagnosis," he said. "We all learn it, but as we get expert, we stop doing it." Experienced doctors are so fast at recognizing common medical conditions that we jump to a diagnosis in seconds. And the minute we find a diagnosis that seems to explain the findings, we stop looking for any other explanation. We stop thinking. This simple form of pattern recognition works well for straightforward conditions, but it can be a trap in more complex situations.

Graber and Singh tried to outline the possible ways doctors could improve diagnostic accuracy.[3] Recognizing that so many diagnostic errors are cognitive in nature, they grouped the possible interventions into three broad categories: increasing knowledge, getting help, and sharpening the thinking process itself.

Increasing knowledge is the traditional manner of bettering ourselves in medicine. The years of medical training, the licensing exams, the recertification process—these are the brute-force ways in which we doctors pound more facts into our heads. In general, this is reasonably successful (it's how we all became doctors, after all), but it's limited by how much stuff you can pack into a given brain.

There are many programs to increase knowledge, but the ones that work best target specific areas and involve intensive training. Periodically, my hospital—and most health organizations—will turn its attention to a single hot-button issue. A few years back, we had an all-hands-on-deck effort to improve the diagnosis of depression. There were workshops and programs and task forces and quality-improvement projects. At times it was overwhelming, but it did significantly raise the profile of depression diagnosis and treatment. Another time there was a similarly intense focus on diagnosing hospital-acquired infections. Another time it was a major initiative toward increasing the accuracy of every patient's medication list.

All of these are valuable initiatives directed at important clinical conditions. It's probably true that our patients benefited, but it's always difficult to prove this. You have to weigh the benefits against the costs in money and time, and also consider what falls by the wayside when everyone converges on one high-profile issue.

Even with the benefits, I'm always left with mixed feelings after each of these full-frontal onslaughts. It's as though we focus the microscope lens of our medical practice on one narrow sliver of medicine, briefly but intensely.

For the moment, you become an expert in that one disease. It's in the differential diagnosis for every single patient you see for the next few months. It's the super-number-one priority in everyone's daily life until it starts to fade into the background. Then some other "quality-improvement project" puts a bee in everyone's bonnet and we've completely forgotten about the first one.

It's not possible to practice medicine that way. You can't keep lasering in on this issue and then that issue and then that one over there. It's discombobulating and ultimately exhausting. The field is just too vast—especially in primary care, where every possible malady of every possible organ is fair game. You can't know—and tackle—*everything* in medicine.

Recognizing the impossibility of knowing everything, Graber and Singh recommend "getting help" as another approach to reduce diagnostic error. Getting a second opinion is something that patients often do, but doctors and nurses can do it too. Curbsiding a colleague with a question is common practice but we could also pursue a formal second opinion the same way patients do. The caveat, though, is that a second opinion is just that—another opinion. While second opinions can help clarify, they can just as easily muddy the waters. And of course, any opinion also has the potential to introduce errors into the situation.

Sharpening the thinking process—the third option—is a much tougher nut to crack. I'll delve into this more in chapters 5 and 15, but even a relatively straightforward case can illustrate the wide range of diagnostic thinking techniques that clinicians can use.

A 57-year-old patient of mine once came to see me about tingling in her hands. She had mild hypertension and elevated cholesterol but was otherwise healthy. Her symptoms weren't exactly in the classic distribution of carpal tunnel syndrome (thumb and first two fingers), but most primary care doctors stick with the dictum—initially, at least—that common things happen commonly. Experience has taught us that an atypical presentation of a common illness is far more likely than a rare illness. (As they say in medical school, "If you hear hoofbeats, think of a horse, not a zebra.") So even if her symptoms didn't fit the textbook exactly, it still was much more likely that she had carpal tunnel syndrome (or some benign variant thereof) than multiple sclerosis or stroke.

I told her to purchase over-the-counter wrist splints, take some ibuprofen, and come back if her condition didn't improve in a few weeks—a fairly standard primary-care response. Looking more critically at my diagnostic process, I know that I did not enumerate a differential diagnosis in the chart. I probably jotted something along the lines of "no red flag signs, most likely carpal tunnel syndrome." If my chart were analyzed by researchers like Graber and

Singh, I'd be dinged for not documenting an explicit differential diagnosis. Of course I'd actually done one in my head, unconsciously, as I interviewed and examined her, mentally eliminating diagnoses that seemed unlikely.

I also knew that the stakes were low; that is, I didn't worry about her dropping dead within a week from a missed diagnosis. I could have ordered electrodiagnostic studies to document carpal tunnel syndrome, but that didn't seem worthwhile. If her symptoms got better within a week or two of her wearing wrist splints, frankly, that's good enough for primary care. And if they didn't, well, then, maybe that would be the time to start ordering tests.

Well, my patient wasn't so happy with my wait-and-see approach, so she promptly saw another doctor, who happened to be a cardiologist. He immediately sent her for electrodiagnostic studies, but he also ordered a nuclear stress test, an echocardiogram, venous dopplers of her legs to look for blood clots, and an arterial-brachial index test to evaluate for arterial disease—all of which were normal.

When she brought me the stack of tests at our next visit some months later, I was floored at the extensive workup she'd received. To me, none of the additional cardiac and vascular tests were indicated. The most charitable explanation I could think of was that yes, sometimes heart disease can present with pain that radiates to the left arm and hand, and yes, this patient's hypertension and cholesterol put her at risk for heart disease. But that was an enormous stretch, given her symptoms of tingling in *both* hands. The least charitable explanation was that the doctor took a look at her insurance and ordered every feasible, billable test. The middle-of-the-road explanation is that when you are a hammer, everything looks like a nail. If you are a cardiologist, any blip of physiology makes you think of the heart and the vascular system.

Still, I wondered about our diagnostic approaches and which of us—if any—was making an error. The cardiologist *did* order the appropriate test for carpal tunnel syndrome. The electrodiagnostic study, incidentally, came out negative; the patient did not have carpal tunnel syndrome, or at least not to any significant degree. So my diagnosis had been wrong. Of course, her hand tingling had improved after using the wrist splints, so maybe I'd been right. Or her hand tingling improved *despite* the wrist splints, so maybe I'd been wrong.

When I put our two approaches to Hardeep Singh, he described it as "the tension between under-diagnosis and over-testing." With my wait-and-see approach, I was running the risk of missing the diagnosis. With the cardiologist's order-every-test-in-the-book approach, he exposed the patient to the risks of over-testing, which include false positives, harms from the tests, and whopping medical bills. "This pendulum of under- and over-testing is what we experience as physicians every day and there are several factors that make physicians swing from one end to the other," Singh said. "Some of us are more tolerant of uncertainty than others. The cardiologist likely doesn't manage uncertainty well, but there could be other reasons he pushed for all those tests, including just giving reassurance to the patient."

In textbooks, diagnoses exist as pristine, self-contained entities, with crisply itemized criteria and clearly enunciated testing strategies. In real medicine, however, uncertainty reigns. Symptoms can be vague, or patients may exhibit only a select few of the symptoms of a particular diagnosis. Patients' symptoms can overlap with a dozen other diagnoses and they can evolve and change over time. Additionally, symptoms can be obscured, such as a fever being masked because the patient took acetaminophen. Nailing a diagnosis amid all this uncertainty has been described as trying to find a "snowball in a blizzard."

If making a diagnosis is tough due to uncertainty, teasing out diagnostic *error* in this ocean of uncertainty is downright daunting. Did a doctor make a mistake in diagnosis, or was she just navigating reasonable uncertainty? This task is made even harder because most research in diagnostic error is done using the EMR. Doctors are forced to select a specific diagnosis code, dictated, of course, by billing purposes. Insurance companies reimburse for diagnoses, not for uncertainty. So there is no legitimate place in the EMR to indicate uncertainty.

Uncertainty also segues into the all-important issue of *context*. Primary care doctors and cardiologists practice in starkly different contexts. As a primary care doc, I take care of everyone from the worried well to the truly sick; there is no filter in my practice. This is one of the things that I love about primary care, but my front-and-center task, then, is to separate out the aches and pains of daily life—of which there are many!—from the graver conditions that require more urgent intervention. This dizzying range of variation means that my practice is awash in uncertainty.

A cardiologist, however, has a practice that has already been filtered. A patient is referred to a cardiologist generally because another doctor strongly suspects heart disease. The amount of uncertainty is therefore much less. There might, then, be value in running an extensive panel of tests on these patients because the baseline prevalence of cardiac disease is so much higher.

By contrast, if I did that same panel of tests on my primary care patients, I'd easily make a host of diagnostic errors. In a group of patients whose illness severity is "diluted out" by all the 18-year-olds with acne and the 35-year-olds with tendinitis, the overall rate of heart disease will be much lower. Any positive results on those tests could very well be false positives.

When my patient came to me with tingling in her hands, I didn't know exactly what her diagnosis was, but I suspected that it would end up in the broad category of minor-symptoms-that-usually-get-better-and-don't-cause-serious-harm. While that isn't a standard medical term you'd find in a textbook or in the EMR, it's a useful way of thinking for primary care doctors on the front line. It might not be the best approach, however, for cardiologists or critical-care doctors, who practice in very different environments with different patient populations.

Diagnostic tests—and diagnostic approaches—do not exist in a vacuum. Context and uncertainty always matter. As Jay's story continues, you will see how different doctors, nurses, and family members navigate uncertainty and how interpretations of context can often be conflicting. I'll discuss more about the diagnostic thinking process itself in chapter 5.

# CHAPTER FOUR

# THE FEVER

Three days after his hospitalization for the induction chemotherapy, Jay had his first follow-up appointment with Dr. Everett. While he waited for the doctor, a nurse came to draw labs from the indwelling catheter that sat just below Jay's clavicle. The nurse introduced herself, but by that point, Jay and Tara had met so many people on the medical team that her name didn't stick. She was young—twentysomething—with long brown hair pulled back in a ponytail.

For patients with serious illness, these indwelling catheters are a godsend because they obviate the need for constant needlesticks for drawing blood, and they can last for several weeks, even months (as opposed to regular IVs, which have to be changed every few days and so swiftly "use up" all the good veins).

The nurse cleaned the ports of Jay's indwelling catheter with alcohol before readying the Vacutainer, the plastic attachment that allows blood to be extracted from the catheter directly into the blood tubes. Jay sat on the exam table chatting with the nurse, while Tara leaned back in an armchair across from him, thumbing through a medical journal. "Well, that port of yours doesn't seem to be working," the nurse was saying to Jay. Tara looked up to see the nurse struggling to affix the Vacutainer onto one of the three ports that emerged from the catheter. Tara noticed that the attachments on the ports were blue. The nurse must have changed them, because they'd been white at home. The Vacutainer that the nurse was pressing onto the port attachment didn't seem to take, because it popped right out into her gloved hand.

Jay kept up the friendly chatter as he did for all the medical folks who crossed his path, asking the nurse how long she'd been in her job, how she liked it, where she was from. The Vacutainer popped off once again, and the nurse again caught it in her hand. Tara sensed that the nurse was getting frazzled from the uncooperativeness of Jay's catheter. There was a lot to juggle with all the ports, the attachments, the blood tubes, and the Vacutainer.

The nurse tried a third time, attempting to twist on the Vacutainer, corkscrew-like. It propelled off with even more momentum, landing on the table next to Jay, on the clean white exam paper that pulls out fresh for each patient. The nurse scooped it up and reattached it to the port. This time, thankfully, it took.

Tara watched the nurse insert the familiar tubes, one by one, into the Vacutainer—the blue-top tube, the red-top, the speckle-top, the purple-top, the black-top. The routine was so second nature to her, everything from the polystyrene crispness of the tubes to the automaticity of knowing which tubes were needed for which particular blood tests to the exact calibration of pressure required to breach the rubber tops with the Vacutainer's hidden inner needle. By this point in her nursing career Tara had probably filled tubes with blood more times than she'd brushed her own teeth.

Yet, it was absolutely surreal for her to see *Jay's* blood lap scarlet into these tubes. Everything familiar now seemed bizarrely foreign, the way a low-resolution video casts only an approximation of real life. No matter how many pixels were stitched together, this couldn't really be Jay sitting on the table with a foot-long catheter connecting his insides to the outside. This couldn't be Jay dangling his legs from the exam table, eliciting the characteristic clinical crinkle of the white paper with even the slightest fidget. This couldn't be Jay—her Jay—already evincing the weariness of a professional patient, despite his ever-ready kind word even for the cleaning crew. It was hardly seven weeks since he'd been Hula-Hooping in their basement, and the exhaustion lines in his face were etched as though they'd been there for decades.

Tara kept wanting to adjust the focus, jiggle the wires, crumple more foil on the rabbit ears, anything to refocus the picture to what things were *supposed* to look like. She and Jay were supposed to be groaning about turning forty and about the unending dramas of teenagers. They were supposed to be stressing about whether they could swing a mortgage for the house they'd been eyeing and how best to balance saving for college versus saving for retirement. They were supposed to be getting ribbings from their kids about receding hairlines, expanding waistlines, and misplaced reading glasses. They *weren't* supposed to be watching Jay's blood spill with mournful diligence into tube after tube after tube.

The nurse finished off by flushing the ports of the catheter with saline (to prevent blood clotting within the narrow tubing). She disconnected the Vacutainer, disposed of it in the sharps bin, and gathered the tubes of blood to send to the lab. Dr. Everett came in and examined Jay. He felt that Jay was doing reasonably well after the induction chemo. Before they could schedule the next round of treatment, though, Jay would need a few weeks to fully recover from this intensive blast of chemo. Jay and Tara needed to watch carefully for even the slightest hint of infection because Jay's bone marrow had been razed to the ground. He was now facing the wide world of pathogens, immunologically naked. Luckily, the human body has a handy alarm system for infection—body temperature. "The most important thing," Dr. Everett stressed to them, "is that Jay needs to come to the hospital *when* the fever begins. Not *if*."

As the doctor predicted, the "when" of the fever began the very next day, Saturday. "Ok, need some positive prayers," Jay wrote that morning on his blog. "My temp is at 99.2 which is higher than my usual 97–98. If I spike to 100.5 I have to go to the hospital to get IV antibiotics. I am going to do some meditation and some praying that it turns around and comes down."

Jay's prayers and meditation did not assuage the mercury. By midday the temperature was 99.9. Tara arrived home after her overnight shift in the ER and surveyed Jay for any localizing signs of infection—cough, rash, vomiting, worsening diarrhea, burning with urination—but he had none.

Tara napped fitfully during the afternoon, checking on Jay every hour or so. The fever hovered up and down, but by 9 p.m. that evening it hit 100.5. Jay and Tara bundled into the car and drove straight to the hospital. The balm of the warm July day was hardly noticeable to them—Tara ramrod straight in the driver seat, rigidly focused on the road, Jay shivering despite his sweatshirt.

On admission to the bone marrow transplant unit (BMTU) Jay's temperature had jumped to 101.5 and now he had shaking chills. The team instituted the standard "fever workup"—chest X-ray, lab tests, blood cultures, urine cultures—and began broad-spectrum antibiotics plus IV saline for hydration. Tara requested that he be hooked up to a telemetry heart monitor—a continuous EKG—because of his previous episodes of fainting. The overnight heme-onc fellow, Dr. Amir, ordered a dose of Demerol—a strong opioid—to control Jay's chills.

"Been up most of the night," Jay wrote at 3:00 a.m. "Starting to feel a little better but can't sleep. We'll see what happens. They should be taking my vitals around 4:00. I think my heart rate dropped when I had to go to the bathroom. This is really annoying, but it is what it is. Guess I can't do anything the easy way!"

The next day, though, Jay felt worse. His fever raged and his appetite soured. An ache in his stomach made it impossible to find a comfortable position. "Wow, I am feeling like garbage," he wrote on that Sunday morning. "This fever is really hot and kicking my butt." His platelets plummeted and he required platelet transfusions to ward off life-threatening bleeding.

"My belly feels full," he confided to Tara. She cast a clinical eye over Jay, and his abdomen did appear slightly distended. His feet seemed a little puffier to her, and the urinal at his bedside did not appear to be filling at the rate that it had been the night before. Tara was clear, though, that she was present as a family member and not as Jay's nurse. She'd certainly witnessed the too-many-cooks phenomenon when family members with medical experience intervened in their loved one's care. Even well-meaning efforts could have disastrous outcomes.

Tara limited herself simply to alerting Jay's nurse of her observations. The nurse was an older white man, and Tara wondered if nursing had been a second career for him. He didn't seem to react with the clinical reflex that was a hallmark of experienced nurses. His assessment of Jay's condition seemed cursory, but Tara didn't want to interfere. Her main concern was about the catheter that was still sitting in Jay's chest while his body burned with fever.

Any indwelling catheter is a potential source of infection. Normally, our twenty square feet of skin keep the outside world safely on the outside. A catheter, however, can act as an express highway for bacteria to venture inside, which is why scrupulous handling is required. Tara winced as she remembered the Vacutainer that had slipped onto the exam table two days earlier. Sure, the white paper was clean. But it wasn't sterile.

The standard rule is that if a patient appears to have an infection, you immediately "pull the line." Even if it looks perfectly clean, it could still be a conduit for infection. No one wants to remove an indwelling catheter unnecessarily, though, because inserting one is not a minor procedure. (Whereas the typical central lines of checklist fame can be inserted at the bedside, indwelling catheters for chemotherapy are surgically implanted in the operating room.) So you don't want to remove an indwelling catheter willy-nilly. But if you think the catheter could be the source of infection, it has to be pulled, no matter what.

All day Sunday, Jay complained about his stomach bothering him. He continued to have a fever, and Tara couldn't figure out why they hadn't pulled the catheter. Midday, the nurse informed Jay of the preliminary results of his blood cultures. "There's all sorts of stuff growing in there," he said. Finding a mix of organisms in a culture rather than a single organism suggests contamination. They'd have to let the cultures grow until the organisms could be identified to see whether they represented true pathogens or just random contaminants. That would take another twenty-four hours.

Still, Jay was continually febrile, despite the antibiotics. And his bone marrow was shot, so his defenses against infection were minimal. Those two facts should be reason enough, Tara thought, to pull the line. But all day

Sunday the catheter remained in use—for fluids, for blood transfusions, for drawing blood samples.

Like all hospitalized patients, Jay had been given an incentive spirometer to help bolster lung capacity. Patients blow into a tube and attempt to keep a plastic ball afloat for as long as possible. But Jay could hardly manage a puff. The ball sat limply at the base. "I can't take a deep breath," he told Tara. "My belly is so full."

During the night his breathing was so noisy that it woke Tara several times. She mentioned this to the overnight nurse, who said this was from the fever. Tara also pointed out that Jay's urine output seemed to be decreasing. The nurse said this was also from the fever.

The next morning, Monday, Jay's feet were more swollen and in Tara's opinion he seemed to be working harder to breathe. She was also increasingly concerned about his *I*'s and *O*'s.

*I*'s and *O*'s stand for *in*'s and *out*'s, and if there's one thing that nurses keep track of scrupulously, probably even in their sleep, it's *I*'s and *O*'s. The amount of fluid going in and the amount going out need to be assiduously measured and they need to be balanced. Too little fluid in and the patient could be dehydrated; too much fluid in and the patient could be overloaded. At the other end, too little fluid coming out and the patient could be in renal failure; too much fluid coming out and the patient could be overmedicated with diuretics. Keeping track of *I*'s and *O*'s is a critical nursing task.

Tara watched the amount of urine accumulating in Jay's urinal and it definitely seemed lower than the day before. IV fluids were still running full force into his body through the catheter, but if his kidneys weren't able to keep up, the fluid could start accumulating in his legs, lungs, and abdomen. Tara informed the day nurse, a soft-spoken woman of Indian descent, about her concerns regarding the imbalanced *I*'s and *O*'s. But the nurse didn't seem to react to this information. She didn't whip out her stethoscope to listen for crackles in Jay's lungs or press on his calves to check for pitting edema of the soft tissues. Tara recalled the nurse just staring back at her, blinking robotically, "like one of those characters in a cartoon."

Later that morning, the bacteria in Jay's blood cultures were identified as MRSA—methicillin-resistant staph aureus. This was both terrifying and relieving for Tara. Terrifying, because blood-borne infections with MRSA are dire, but also relieving, because now there was an explanation for Jay's fever and the treatment could be tailored to that.

Once MRSA had been confirmed, of course, there was no choice but to pull the line. However, because Jay's platelets were still low, he would need additional platelet transfusions to effectively stanch the bleeding in the wake of the catheter's removal. Plus Jay was still anemic, so he needed a regular (red-cell) blood transfusion as well. This could take hours.

Tara steamed inwardly as she watched the nurse administer the blood products on her own. Proper protocol requires *two* nurses to be present at the beginning of any blood transfusion so that identity and blood type can be meticulously crosschecked. But at this point, she was too exhausted to complain. She'd hardly slept in thirty-six hours and felt like the staff was starting to tune her out. They'd probably already pegged her as one of those "difficult" family members who just made their work harder.

Dr. Chowdury, the heme-onc fellow, came by on her rounds, and Tara felt instant relief at seeing her, remembering how attentive she'd been during Jay's admission the previous week. Tara unloaded her pent-up concerns: Jay's difficulty breathing, the fullness in his abdomen, the edema in his feet, the decreased urine output. Dr. Chowdury listened carefully and examined Jay. Jay pointed to his right chest, saying that it was hurting there now. Dr. Chowdury ordered a chest X-ray, as well as an abdominal X-ray.

There was a different hematology attending on the ward this week—Dr. Mueller—who came by shortly thereafter. In Tara's recollection, Dr. Mueller had the rosy cheeks and portly build of a female Santa Claus. But she wasn't exactly jolly. Her tone was rather terse when Tara again related her concerns. Even though Dr. Chowdury had listened attentively, Tara was well aware that the attending physician was ultimately in charge, so it mattered what Dr. Mueller thought.

Dr. Mueller listened to Jay's lungs and commented that she heard crackles at the right base. Crackles could signify a pneumonia, but they could also represent fluid overload. The X-ray would help distinguish between those two possibilities. Tara noticed that Dr. Mueller did not examine Jay's abdomen, even though Jay had been complaining of right-sided abdominal pain. Jay had sported six-pack abs his entire life, so what might seem like a little middle-age flab on some people, Tara knew, was abnormal. For Jay, this was true distention.

Tara waited anxiously for the X-ray results, but they turned out to be unhelpful. There was no specific pneumonia or fluid buildup that could explain Jay's increased work of breathing. Tara knew that the diagnostic process was rarely straightforward, especially in patients whose immune systems had been pummeled by leukemia and then further trammeled by chemotherapy. Still, something was going on, and something needed to be done. Jay was now talking in whispers because it was too hard to speak at a normal volume.

"Look at how hard he is working," Tara pointed out to the nurse.

"It's from the chemo," the nurse replied.

"Could we please start him on oxygen?" Tara asked.

"He doesn't need it," the nurse said, pointing at the oxygen saturation monitor, which showed his levels to be in the normal range, though edging down toward the lower range of normal.

Tara was losing her patience. "His respiratory rate is in the thirties," she said, pointing at Jay's heaving chest. "And his heart rate is in the 120s to 130s. Sustained! He can't keep up like this." She recalled the nurse just standing there, looking at her with that same cartoon-character blank look. Tara had vowed not to interfere with Jay's actual medical care, but she just couldn't take it any longer. She stared straight at the nurse and said firmly, "Go get me a nasal cannula." The nurse complied and returned shortly thereafter with the oxygen setup.

Later in the day, a chatty email arrived from their daughter Sasha in China. "I ate mushrooms and some beef and fish and a lot of fried rice. And some fried stuff (I'm gonna learn how to make it today). It's actually pretty good food, I am going to miss it, and tea, when I get home." She was teaching English at an orphanage, supplementing the lessons with Frisbee and basketball for the kids. She'd hiked a glacier-covered mountain, subjected herself to the rigors of Tibetan dancing, and was trying her level best to follow the Chinese soap operas that her host family favored. Her visit to a monastery left such an impression that she bought a scroll of Chinese prayers to give to her father and had been sketching the monks deep in meditation. "I hope you know I am going to be past exhausted when I get home. It's a 12-hour time change. I'll want to sleeeep in bed for a while. And eat steak. And Papa's potatoes . . ."

Her optimism and excitement bubbled through, almost as though she were standing there right next to them. Sasha still did not know that her father was in the hospital, or even that he'd been diagnosed with leukemia. She didn't know that Jay had a fever and was struggling to breathe. But her letter brought a burst of warmth into the gray hospital room. Tears ran down Jay's cheeks as Tara read the letter aloud. "I'm so . . . proud of her," he whispered between gasps for breath.

It still weighed on Tara and Jay that they hadn't disclosed to Sasha all they were struggling with. But they accepted this burden, even gladly, because they knew they'd enabled her to enjoy this once-in-lifetime experience to its fullest. The pain would come—there was no way around it—but they could protect their child for a little bit longer.

CHAPTER FIVE

# DIAGNOSTIC THINKING

Medical shows on TV are popular because we are enraptured by the brilliant doctor who plucks an esoteric diagnosis out of the hat, based on some obscure clinical detail and a keen memory for arcane facts. When we ourselves are patients, however, we prefer decidedly less drama. We like it when the diagnosis is straightforward and reassuringly boring. In real life nobody wants to be a diagnostic puzzle or a cliffhanger ending.

As we can see with Jay, real life in medicine is immensely complicated. Textbook logic for making a diagnosis falls apart in the messy world of human physiology, rendering medicine even less akin to the aviation industry. Even when we think we have a culprit—in Jay's case, the MRSA bacteria growing in his blood—there is still uncertainty. Jay's condition was worsening despite antibiotics for MRSA. Was the problem ineffective treatment? Delayed treatment? Perhaps there were other diagnoses brewing alongside the MRSA infection?

It was particularly notable that Jay was short of breath and remained febrile. Shortness of breath has many possible explanations, but in the presence of a fever, pneumonia is the prime contender. His chest X-ray was reported as "negative" for pneumonia, but this illustrates one of the challenges of making an accurate diagnosis. Does a negative chest X-ray mean that a patient does *not* have pneumonia?

As always, context counts. A negative chest X-ray could reasonably rule out a pneumonia in a healthy person with a mild cough sitting comfortably in a doctor's office. But in the context of a critically ill, febrile, immunocompromised patient in a hospital ward who is struggling to breathe, a negative chest X-ray assumes a different meaning, or several meanings. It could represent a false negative; that is, the pneumonia exists, but the X-ray did not show it. Or a negative X-ray report could mean that the radiologist made an error when reading the film, but the X-ray actually did show a pneumonia. Alternatively, it could be that an X-ray is the wrong test to diagnose pneumonia in this context; an X-ray might simply be incapable of picking up a pneumonia in a patient whose devastated immune system can't gin up the normal inflammatory response that creates the typical X-ray findings.

Patients often assume that tests such as X-rays are objective, like calculators: put in the numbers and the correct answer will be spit out. Reading X-rays, however, is a learned, cognitive skill done by humans, who have to render subjective decisions about what constitutes normal and what constitutes pathology. Sometimes a pneumonia on a chest X-ray is blindingly obvious—an entire chunk of lung is whited-out from inflammation. But often, the radiologic signs of pneumonia are subtle. Countless times I've stared at a patch of haziness on an X-ray until my eyes water, debating whether this vague fuzziness represents a true pneumonia or whether it's just *schmutz* (a word that has migrated seamlessly from Yiddish to official radiologic terminology). A good radiologist spends years staring at films, learning the copious variations that inflammation and infection of the lung tissue can take.

Because X-ray reading is essentially about visual pattern recognition, it's an area in which technology and artificial intelligence is making headway. You teach a doctor to read X-rays by showing her enough examples during her training, and the idea is that you could similarly teach a computer system the same thing by inputting a sufficient number of images. Trial and error should allow the system to learn to distinguish what is pathology from what is *schmutz*.

A group of researchers from California have tried to create such a system by uploading images from 112,120 chest X-rays.[5] These X-rays had been individually labeled as normal or as having up to fourteen abnormalities, including pneumonia. The researchers created an algorithm to analyze the images and with "machine learning" were able to train the system in much the way you'd train a radiology resident. They then tested the system with 420 new X-rays to see how well it did in diagnosing pneumonia. And for fun, they tested it against nine radiologists from esteemed academic institutions, who independently reviewed the same 420 images.

The computerized system did just as well as its human counterparts for ten of the fourteen pulmonary abnormalities, including pneumonia, lung masses, and fluid in and around the lungs (the radiologists edged out the system for emphysema, hiatal hernia, and enlarged heart). Furthermore, it was able to evaluate the 420 X-rays in 1.5 minutes, whereas the humans took an average of 240 minutes. It isn't necessarily surprising that the computerized system did so well—and didn't need coffee or bathroom breaks—since accurate pattern recognition relates to the sheer amount of experience in seeing prior patterns. With a computerized system, you can take the foie gras approach and endlessly cram in the images. Unlike with a goose—or a radiology resident, for that matter—you won't get squawks, ruptured intestines, or "Oh, it's 6 p.m., I gotta run."

Success with visual pattern recognition has sparked interest in using artificial intelligence and computerized algorithms to improve diagnostic accuracy for a wide variety of medical conditions. For straightforward clinical situations, such as whether an ankle injury requires an X-ray to distinguish a sprain from a fracture, it's relatively easy to create an algorithm. But it's a whole other can of worms to teach a computer to make a diagnosis when a patient presents with a vague symptom like "My stomach hurts" or "I'm feeling more tired these days."

Improving the grand diagnostic process is something of a holy grail for researchers in this field. Wouldn't it be great to have a system in which you could enter the patient's symptoms, and the program would create an accurate differential diagnosis? It would include all the rare diseases that fallible humans tend to forget but, of course, eliminate the ones that are too far out in left field. It would generate an intelligent road map for a thorough—but not reckless—workup. It would take into account cost efficiency and clinical context and assiduously avoid both false-positive and false-negative errors. Holy grail, indeed!

Several diagnostic tools have been created with this goal in mind, and a few of them are out there in practice: ISABEL, VisualDx, and DXplain ("Dx" is medical shorthand for diagnosis). A review that analyzed all the published studies about these programs came to mixed conclusions.[2] Researchers didn't find compelling evidence to make a wholesale recommendation for doctors to use them but did say that they had the potential to be of assistance. I spent an afternoon trying out these systems when I was supervising in our walk-in clinic. Each time a resident or student presented a case, I'd enter the symptoms into the system. Before I pressed "submit," we'd come up with our own differential diagnosis and then compare our results to the computer. For the cases that were straightforward, the system was far too laborious; our minds were much faster and more efficient. But then we got a case that represented a diagnostic dilemma. Perfect for testing out the system.

The case involved a young, healthy woman in her early twenties who was experiencing episodes of rapid heart rate and shortness of breath. She'd previously played on sports teams but was now too fatigued to do so. Financial difficulties had recently forced her family to move into a cramped basement apartment. She disliked it intensely and felt very anxious whenever she was alone in the apartment.

She'd already stayed overnight in the hospital after an ER visit and the major cardiac causes had been ruled out. The cardiologists felt it was anxiety that was making her heart race, and when they gave her a beta-blocker to slow the heart rate, she felt better, though not completely.

As soon as my team and I began typing in the symptoms, we realized just how formidable it is to quantify the diagnostic process. Entering "tachycardia" and "dyspnea" (racing heart and shortness of breath) brought up a voluminous list of possible diagnoses. The system was casting a wide net so that it wouldn't miss anything, but we humans wouldn't have wasted an iota of mental effort on a good chunk of their diagnoses. For example, the list was headed up by "septic shock"—which of course can present with those symptoms. But when you are evaluating a healthy-appearing woman who is smiling and chatting amiably with you, septic shock would never enter your mind (as opposed to when you are evaluating a patient like Jay, who also had tachycardia and dyspnea). Nor would massive hemorrhage or ruptured aortic aneurysm—two other diagnoses that appeared on the list.

There was no box to type in the "gist" of what this young woman was like. There was no place for context. There was no field to enter psychosocial issues like "financial stress forcing move to claustrophobic, subterranean apartment." I don't fault the system for this, but these limitations highlight the breadth of the elements that enter into the diagnostic process. Furthermore, the system wouldn't be able to consider that a basement apartment might host more mold than an upstairs apartment. Mold causes or exacerbates a host of pulmonary ailments, from asthma to aspergillosis to hypersensitivity pneumonitis, so the system would miss these possibilities.

In reviewing the differential diagnosis list that the system provided for our case, we quickly crossed off the assorted catastrophic conditions that weren't remotely a consideration in a walking, talking, not-prostrate-on-a-gurney patient. The remainder of the list mostly contained things we'd already considered, such as hyperthyroidism and anemia. It did mention a few that we might not have thought about, such as acute porphyria and sodium azide poisoning. Our conclusion was that the system didn't really parallel the manner in which we think about patients, but it could be useful to jog our memories for rarer things.

One of the major criticisms of these computerized diagnosis systems is that they have an incentive to cast their nets as widely as possible. This allows the commercial developers to tout impressive statistics about how frequently the correct diagnosis appears on the list. But in actual clinical practice, doctors have to make real-world trade-offs, especially when it comes to rarer diagnoses that require expensive tests with risks of harm to patients.

We also have to factor in the logistics of the diagnostic workup: How long will it take to get a CT scan? Does the patient's insurance cover an MRI? When is the next available rheumatology appointment? Can the patient take off time from work to get that thyroid scan? There are also patients' preferences that affect the diagnostic process: How aggressive does he want to be? How risk averse is she? What are his financial concerns? All of these real-world considerations play a role in how we do diagnostic workups—all intricacies that do not burden these sleekly insouciant algorithms.

Lastly, there are the practical aspects of real-time use. These systems take time to employ. A doctor would have to, in essence, stop her evaluation of the patient in order to give time to the algorithm. Given how time-crunched medical evaluations are these days, anything that subtracts from the (already limited) direct face time between doctors and patients has to offer proven value.

These systems are impressive works of technology whose role is still evolving. Most likely, they will be resources for complex cases and for teaching. But it is important to keep in mind that simply generating a list of possibilities isn't the same as making the diagnosis. A computer doesn't have to commit. A doctor does. And so does the patient.

For the young woman we were evaluating in the walk-in clinic, most of the workup came back negative. Her chest X-ray and pulmonary function tests were normal. Unlike a computerized algorithm, we still had to do something to help her symptoms. We still had to commit, even in the absence of a specific diagnosis.

The most important diagnostic clue remained the fact that her breathing was better when she was out of the apartment. So whether it was mold in the apartment that was triggering respiratory symptoms or claustrophobia that was causing anxiety, the best treatment we could offer was to help her structure her life to spend more time away from the apartment. She began spending weekends with her aunt and occasional weeknights with friends. On a follow-up visit she said she felt that her symptoms were improving. She was now focusing her energies on saving enough money to eventually move out on her own.

---

Computerized algorithms are one way to try to minimize diagnostic errors. But is there a way to improve how doctors do their own internal algorithms? Is there a way to improve the actual thinking? Refining this overall process of diagnostic reasoning is a more global approach that could potentially improve things in *all* areas of medicine, and it would avoid the pitfalls of the disease-of-the-week approach that many healthcare systems use in tackling medical error.

Mark Graber and Hardeep Singh, the researchers focused on improving diagnostic accuracy, admit that targeting thinking is far more challenging than standard quality-improvement projects such as reducing hospital-acquired infections or screening for depression. Is it an impossible task? "With ten thousand diseases, there is so much uncertainty," Graber admits. "We get it right 90% of the time. That's pretty amazing!" And then he adds slyly, "But can we get it to 95%?"

Nudging the accuracy rate up, rather than attempting to eliminate *all* diagnostic error, seems like a doable prospect. But thinking styles are deeply ingrained and decidedly recalcitrant when commanded to evolve. Our declarations of rationality are routinely undercut by our unconscious biases, not to mention those rascally emotions that we are convinced we retain mastery of. Additionally, our thinking styles are routinely and unceremoniously jolted when we are rushed, pressured, inattentive, or otherwise distracted.

There are times when we cogitate like Kant and other times when we rely on intuition and guesswork like $5 sidewalk psychics. Mental shortcuts abound in our reasoning and our reliance on them is matched only by our chipper unawareness of using them. Such capricious thinking patterns aren't as amenable to typical patient-safety checklists or aviation-style standardization.

Furthermore, it is not clear how such research could even be done. As Semmelweis, Nightingale, and Pronovost all demonstrated, you need to be able to measure the problem, apply an intervention, and then track the results with meaningful real-world outcomes. How would you take even the first step with regard to diagnostic reasoning? There isn't a thought-o-meter that researchers can seamlessly slip into our cerebral gyri to measure our reasoning process in all its fits of brilliance and banality. If asked, most of us probably couldn't even describe how we think. So while it makes intuitive sense to work on the thinking process, doing the actual research is no picnic. As a result, data in this field are notably sparse.

Nevertheless, since the thought process is the source of most diagnostic error, there is still value in pursuing this avenue. It is especially beneficial in the early years of medical school and nursing school, as this is when diagnostic "habits" are formed. And even for established clinicians, there is probably at least some value in thinking about how we think. Even if only modestly effective, it is likely the truest way to decrease diagnostic error.

There are several techniques that can be used to hone our diagnostic thinking process, and they share in common the idea of resisting the urge to jump to an easy conclusion. They start with Graber's dictum about the "discipline of the differential diagnosis." Every time doctors evaluate patients, they should force themselves to consider a range of possibilities before homing in on a single one. The very act of considering alternatives opens up the mind to, well, alternatives. You can't get to a particular diagnosis if you never actually consider it.

So how do you do this in real time? As soon as a first diagnosis is entertained, the doctor (and the patient) should ask, "Could it be anything else?"—Graber and Singh call this the "universal antidote" to diagnostic error—and then keep asking it. A cough, for example, may seem like a standard viral URI (upper respiratory infection) at first blush, but what else could it be? Sinusitis, bronchitis, influenza, and pneumonia all have a cough component. Gastric reflux can present with a cough, as can asthma. A cough could also be a sign of congestive heart failure or a side effect of ACE inhibitors (a class of blood pressure medications). A cough could signify tuberculosis or lung cancer. It might be emphysema or pertussis (whooping cough). A cough could be caused by environmental irritants such as mold, or by accidentally inhaling objects that are best left outside the body.

What *else* could it be? Well, there are a host of less common conditions that can present with cough, such as sarcoidosis, interstitial lung disease, vascular malformations, or blood clots in the lung. And then there are the rare diseases such as amyloidosis, relapsing polychondritis, granulomatosis with polyangiitis, and psychogenic cough. And the even rarer conditions like syngamosis, pulmonary Langerhans cell histiocytosis, and tracheobronchopathia osteochondroplastica.

Or maybe the cough is just plain old post-nasal drip.

While it isn't necessary to hoof it as far as tracheobronchopathia osteochondroplastica for the average patient with a cough, the point is that the more you ask yourself, "What else could it be?" the more ideas you come up with. The vast majority of coughs will fall into the first few tiers of the differential, but it's still important to think beyond. As attendings intone—ad infinitum—to medical students on rounds, "No one ever made the diagnosis of sarcoidosis without first considering sarcoidosis in the differential." The nice thing about the what-else-could-it-be strategy is that it's straightforward and its logic fits naturally with the whole idea of the differential diagnosis.

There are some variations on this strategy. Considering the consequences of a missed diagnosis of a more severe illness is another way to challenge your thinking. Yes, most coughs in a typical primary care setting flower in the URI/bronchitis/sinusitis garden and will get better on their own no matter what you do or don't do. But what if the cough is the harbinger of a lung cancer? Or a blood clot? Missing these could be devastating, even deadly, so even though they are far less frequent, we always need to be sure we've thought about these severe diagnoses and then rallied the data that would exclude them.

When I am reviewing a case with students or interns, I push them to give a full differential, not just jump out with the one diagnosis that seems obvious. After they've provided their list, I'll ask the two golden questions: "What else could it be?" and "Is there anything that we can't afford to miss?"

The hard part is remembering to do this for myself. When I'm rushing through a busy day, backlogged with patients and overwhelmed with the never-ending EMR minutiae, this discipline melts away faster than the smooth talk from a drug rep. If it walks like a URI and quacks like a URI, I'll pretty quickly chalk up that cough to a URI without rigorously questioning myself. How many diagnostic errors have I made by doing this? Unfortunately, I'll never know.

Another cognitive trick is to focus on the data that *don't* fit your presumptive diagnosis. If I'm making the diagnosis of URI in a patient with a cough who also has a rash, I should expend a neuron or two on the fact that rash is not usually associated with a URI. That would force me to reconsider my diagnosis. Maybe it's something other than a URI, such as infection with parvovirus B19 or Epstein-Barr virus. Or maybe the patient has two different things going on. Patients with URIs, after all, are allowed to also have eczema. Or maybe the patient took a medication to treat the URI and had an allergic reaction to it.

These questions and exercises designed to sharpen diagnostic thinking have the makings of—you guessed it—a checklist! Mark Graber, along with John Ely and Pat Croskerry, explored the idea of checklists for diagnosis and recognized that you really need two distinct types of checklists—one for content and one for process.[3] Content checklists could be the computerized algorithms mentioned earlier that are tailored to the specific patient data that you enter or they could just be plain old lists. Ely, a family physician in Iowa, developed a convenient set of lists for outpatient use.[4] He categorized the forty-six most common complaints in outpatient medicine (dizziness, abdominal/pelvic pain, diarrhea, headache, insomnia, etc.) and then listed a dozen or two of the most common causes, with a few tricky ones labeled "commonly missed" and a few serious ones labeled "do not miss." It's a quick way for a doctor to run down a list and make sure she hasn't missed anything.

By contrast, *process* checklists review the thought process, looking for biases and shortcuts that might undercut diagnostic accuracy. Graber, Singh, and colleagues created a process checklist that includes the standard "What else could it be?" and "What can I not afford to miss?" but also asks some other interesting questions that can affect accuracy. Did I simply accept the first diagnosis that came to mind? Did someone else—patient, colleague—already put on a diagnostic label that's biasing me? Was the patient recently evaluated for the same complaint? Am I distracted or overtired right now? Is this a patient that I don't like for some reason? Is this a patient I like too much (family member, friend, colleague)?[5]

The point of these questions is to make you stop and think. For complex cases in which things don't make sense, you can take the extra step and do a full-fledged "diagnostic timeout," similar to the standard timeout procedure before starting surgery. This is especially helpful when existing diagnoses don't quite add up. I have a patient whose chart listed rheumatoid arthritis (RA) in every note since the Paleolithic era. When I took over her care from a departing doctor, I dutifully listed RA in every one of *my* notes. Over the years, though, it slowly dawned on me that she never actually experienced any specific symptoms of RA (swollen, tender joints in a symmetrical distribution associated with significant morning stiffness). One day I finally took a diagnostic timeout and dug back through her voluminous chart. After some deep hunting, I found the workup from years earlier in which two classic blood tests for RA were "positive." That, alongside some nonspecific aches and pains, was how the diagnosis was implanted in her chart. It became entrenched and every subsequent doctor repeated the gospel until it was simply a fact of her medical history. But the truth was that she did not actually have rheumatoid arthritis—those initial blood tests were likely false positives. Diagnoses do indeed evolve over time; this one took a decade to figure out.

Diagnostic checklists, however, are harder to implement than other checklists. Presurgical checklists consist mostly of clear-cut, tangible items: Did we check the patient's name? The surgical site? They take one second to answer and then you are done and can move on. Well, how do you know when a thought is done? How do you know when to end the "what else could it be" line of thinking? How do you decide whether your fatigue or distraction are significant enough to impair your thinking (given that everyone is exhausted and that interruptions are incessant)?

Additionally, most pre-surgical (and pre-flight) checklists are performed aloud with other people. Not so in diagnosis. "Diagnosis is usually silent, lonely work," write Ely, Graber, and Croskerry. "A natural pause point to review the checklist, such as before takeoff or before incision, does not exist in diagnosis, which can stretch over hours, days, or even months."

Many doctors find diagnostic checklists off-putting because they include things that are obvious, even insulting—take a complete history, read the X-ray yourself, take time to reflect. But these authors point out that pilots don't feel insulted running down their checklists or being questioned by their copilots.

They might have initially, but now it's simply part of the job. Importantly, they don't do it only in difficult situations; they do it every time, even when they are flying with the most experienced crews on the most perfect sunny days. Doctors, on the other hand, tend to see value in these checklists—if they do at all—only for the difficult cases and diagnostic conundrums.

When I think honestly about my own practice style as a physician, I recognize—with no small amount of abashment—that my approach is cursory or intuitive far more than I'd want to admit. In the survival mode that most doctors and nurses work in today, it's easy to fall back on snap judgments and obvious diagnoses. Fighting the current to slow down and question my thinking is arduous, especially when I feel like I'm struggling just to keep my head above water most days.

One Monday morning, a patient handed me a note from a pain-management doctor that he was seeing at another institution. In the course of sending out an unnecessarily expansive panel of blood tests, a cortisol level came out slightly low. The doctor had jotted a one-liner for me on a sheet of his prescription paper: "Rule out adrenal insufficiency."

As my patient began updating me on his six other chronic conditions, I surreptitiously pulled up the webpage on adrenal insufficiency. Not that I don't remember every detail of adrenal vagaries, mind you. And, sure, I'd re-memorized it all for my board recertification two years prior, but let's just say that adrenal insufficiency is one of those conditions that resides out on a wobbly, far-flung cortical gyrus.

Adrenal insufficiency is a notoriously knotty topic. The symptoms are both varied and vague. There is primary adrenal insufficiency and secondary adrenal insufficiency. There is acute adrenal insufficiency and chronic adrenal insufficiency. To test for it, I'd have to give the patient a dose of a hormone to stimulate the adrenal gland and then check cortisol levels at zero, thirty, and sixty minutes. There were at least ten variations on how to administer that hormone and even more variations on how to interpret the results. And could I even figure out how to order three separate, timed blood draws? Within a minute, my head was spinning.

While my patient updated me on his back pain, his diabetes, and his GI symptoms, I dug through the fine print to remind myself which way the diurnal variation of cortisol runs: Up in the morning? Down at night? Or vice versa? My patient stacked his fifteen medications on my desk—all of which needed refills, and all of which could interfere with adrenal function and/or adrenal testing. I realized I simply could not sort this all out in the moment.

What I needed was time to think.

I found myself pining for those medical-school Saturdays in the library—endless hours to read and think. Nothing but me, knowledge, and silence, facing off in a tai chi battle of concentration. How I hated those study sessions then, and how I would have given my left adrenal for a few minutes of that now.

But a gazillion EMR fields were demanding attention. Three more charts were waiting in my box. The patient still had two MRI reports and an endoscopy report for me to review, plus a question about prostate testing.

His adrenal insufficiency was swamped by my cerebral insufficiency.

I could tell him I'd review his case later and get back to him. But what "later" were we talking about? My morning session would run overtime by hours—that was a given. There were last week's labs to review, student notes to check, patient calls to return, meds to renew, forms and papers erupting in a Cubist dystopia all over my desk. There would never *be* any "later." ("Later" is a fantasy dreamed up by bureaucrat who've never set foot outside a cubicle.) There was only now.

But if I made any clinical decisions now, they would be haphazard, rife with potential for error. They would be an embarrassment. I finally threw in the towel and scribbled a referral to endocrinology—let *them* deal with it. I hustled my patient out the door and hurried the next person in.

In the pressurized world of contemporary medicine, there is simply no time to think. It certainly doesn't feel like I have time to run through extensive diagnostic checklists, no matter how logical and important they seem. I sometimes feel as though I am racing to cover the bare minimum, sprinting in subsistence-level intellectual mode because that's all that's sustainable. I confess that I harbor a fear of anything "atypical" popping up during a visit. I dread symptoms that don't add up, test results that are contradictory, patients who lug in bagfuls of herbal supplements with instructions to "ask your doctor." If I can't spring to a conclusion in a minute flat, I'm sunk. God help me if their medical history includes Sturge-Weber syndrome or polyarteritis nodosa. I don't even have enough time to type them (or spell them!), much less look them up and remind myself what they are.

So when I think about the reasoned approach that Graber, Singh, and other researchers suggest, I applaud it. I second it. I *yearn* for it. But it's hard to see how it can fit in with the everyday experiences of most doctors and nurses.

A few days after the visit with that patient, I happened on *Core IM*, an internal medicine podcast created by some of my NYU colleagues. One of the hosts mentioned an episode on adrenal insufficiency. "It's one of those topics," he observed, "that's never nailed down fully."

Ah, so maybe I wasn't the only idiot who couldn't iron out adrenal insufficiency on the fly. Maybe I wasn't such a loser for not being able to orient the hypothalamic-pituitary-adrenal axis in the middle of a chaotic clinic session. I listened to the episode and then reread the chapter. With an actual case in hand, the physiology clicked more easily. The next day, I went to work early, opened the patient's chart, and resifted through his data.

I still wanted him to see an endocrinologist, but at least now I didn't feel like I was handing off a mess. I appended my initial note with a more intelligible analysis and called the patient to explain our plan. When I closed out the chart, I felt satisfied with the case for the first time. In retrospect, I realize that I had taken a full-fledged diagnostic timeout, which is what this case required. It felt frankly thrilling to have given medical care at the appropriate level of thoroughness, to have fended off the cutting of corners we're so often forced to employ.

Of course, sorting out this *one* issue for this *one* patient took a full hour outside his visit. I couldn't have pulled it off in the moment, and I can't carve out an extra hour during that nonexistent "later" for every patient with a complex problem. But that's what so many of our patients' diagnoses require—time to think, consider, revisit, reanalyze. From the billing-and-coding perspective, this is supremely inefficient. There's no diagnosis code for "cognitive pandemonium." There's no billing code for "contemplation." But extra time dedicated to thinking—using diagnostic checklists to expand our differential diagnosis as well as to examine our thinking process—could actually be remarkably efficient.

Time to think seems quaint in our metrics-driven, pay-for-performance, throughput-obsessed healthcare system, but we'd make fewer diagnostic errors and surely save money by reducing unnecessary tests and cop-out referrals. I suspect time to think would also make a substantial dent in the demoralization of medical professionals today, but that's a whole other story.

---

Reducing diagnostic error will ultimately require a culture shift in healthcare. We need to reorient how we think as well as the culture that impedes our thinking. According to Singh, this would involve "acknowledging uncertainty and associating humility rather than heroism with our diagnostic decision-making capabilities."[6] There are few diagnoses more rare in the medical species than intellectual humility. There are few allergies more common than that of doctors to uncertainty.

"Overconfidence is an enormous problem," Graber observed to me, "both personal and organizational." We're so sure of our snap-judgment diagnosis that we rarely stop to think about what else it could be, much less whether our thought process was flawed in any way. If we do, it's usually only on a very cursory level.

But Graber also admitted that overconfidence doesn't come about just because we doctors think we're so smart (although that arrogance is certainly a hefty contributor!) but that it also stems from a lack of feedback. If we never hear back from the patient, then we assume everything is fine and that we must have been correct in our diagnosis. That may indeed be the case some of the time. But it's equally plausible that not hearing back means the patient didn't get better and that we were wrong. The patient might have sought care elsewhere and been given the correct diagnosis by a different doctor. Or worse, not hearing back from our patients might mean they've exited stage left thanks to our missteps. But we have no way of knowing.

It was when Graber suggested that doctors ought to have something like "Stump the Chumps" that I knew we were kindred spirits. For more years than I care to admit, I've been inexplicably addicted to the radio show *Car Talk*. Hosted by Tom and Ray Magliozzi, brothers endowed with capacious Boston accents and equally capacious belly laughs, it was a call-in show about automotive repair. Full disclosure: I'm a Manhattanite who doesn't own a car and hopes to remain auto-less till my last terrestrial breath. But there I was, week in and week out, riveted by the discussions of head gaskets and timing belts. The shows were funnier than most TV shows billed as comedy and surprisingly informative (hey, taxis break down occasionally, so even New Yorkers need to know their camshafts from their crankshafts).

Even when the show went off the air, I listened to reruns. Even after Tom sadly passed away, I listened to the podcasts—I was that much of a groupie. It didn't matter that the cars they were talking about were twenty years out of date; there was something ridiculously comforting hearing about the "staff" that included Russian chauffeur Picov Andropov, Greek tailor Euripedes Imenedes, and the white-glove law firm Dewey, Cheetham, and Howe. After particularly aggravating days in the hospital, I turn on the *Car Talk* podcast before I've even hung up my white coat. It works faster than Valium and the only side effect is cackling like a goofball while crossing Twenty-Eighth Street.

So it was an unexpected delight when I interviewed Mark Graber and he—unprompted—brought up *Car Talk* in our conversation. Every few weeks, Tom and Ray would run a segment called "Stump the Chumps" in which they'd bring back a caller from a previous show. They'd replay the original call and review their analysis at the time. Then the caller would tell them how things played out, and Tom and Ray would learn if they'd made the correct automotive diagnosis or not.

Graber's point was that we need something like "Stump the Chumps" in medicine—a regular feature in which patients come back and let us know how they fared and whether we got the diagnosis right. In academic centers, there are M&M ("morbidity and mortality") conferences, but these tend to focus on disasters. And patients—even if they've survived—aren't typically part of the M&M process. In reality, there isn't really any forum—either in academia or private practice—for ongoing feedback from patients in these more ordinary situations. A dose of *Car Talk* for this (and for many a mind-numbing administrative meeting) might be just what the doctor ordered. You never know when you'll need to call upon *Car Talk*'s director of staff bonuses, Xavier Breath, or bungee-jumping instructor, Hugo First.

Sixteen years after the Institute of Medicine published the *To Err Is Human* report, which set the patient-safety movement in motion, it took up the subject of diagnostic error.* The report offered the chilling observation that nearly everyone will experience at least one diagnostic error in their lifetime.[7] It's quite a damning statistic, one that garnered eye-catching news headlines. Of course, not all of these diagnostic errors have significant clinical consequences (misdiagnosing mild arthritis for tendinitis is unlikely to harm anyone, especially since they are treated nearly identically). But many misdiagnoses have the potential to cause significant harm to patients, in addition to squandering prodigious amounts of money.

Refreshingly, the report did not simply point the finger at the incompetence of individual physicians, as both lawsuits and popular media tend to do. Rather, it described a Borgesian healthcare system that seems almost intentionally designed to stymie the diagnostic thought process. It noted that our reimbursement system favors procedures over thoughtful analysis. That is, more revenue is generated if I order an MRI for all of my patients with abdominal pain than if I spend extra time talking with them and sorting out the details.

If I review a case with a colleague to get a second opinion, or call a radiologist to discuss whether a less expensive ultrasound would suffice, that would not be reimbursed in our current system. If I make additional phone calls to

*In that same year, the IOM also changed its name to the National Academy of Medicine and folded into the far less abbreviatable "National Academies of Sciences, Engineering, and Medicine." Like many of my colleagues, though, I retain a soft spot for the more mellifluous "IOM."

a patient after the visit to elicit further clarifying information, that too would be ignored by the billing system.

Talking about reimbursement may reinforce the stereotype that doctors care only about money. But in reality, if something is not reimbursed, it's hard to get it done because there are only so many hours in the day. For time-pressed clinicians, the system makes it faster and easier to simply order MRIs than to think longer and deeper about our patients' cases.

So bravo to the IOM for recognizing that diagnosis can be a team sport, and that time spent analyzing a case is as critically important as tests and procedures. The report explicitly presses insurance companies to reimburse for the cognitive side of medicine and to eliminate the financial distortion that overwhelmingly favors procedures over thinking.

Additionally, there needs to be a mechanism for clinicians to report their own errors without fear of getting sued or reprimanded. Near misses—errors that almost happen, or errors that occur but don't cause harm—represent perhaps the largest trove of information for improving healthcare. Yet medical professionals tend to keep quiet about them, because of both liability fears and the personal shame that accompanies such errors. In chapter 11, I'll examine efforts to address these concerns.

Overall, diagnostic error is far thornier to tackle than errors related to procedures (e.g., putting in central lines) or even medication errors. The sheer number of possible diseases multiplied by infinite human variability makes diagnosis much less amenable to simplistic checklists and rigid algorithms. Real-life clinical medicine never lays out like the neat bullet points of task-force reports, no matter how expert or well-meaning the authors are.

There's an old adage that 90% of diagnoses are made just by taking a patient's history. This probably isn't 100% accurate, but it's pretty darn close. Patients and their families are arguably the truest experts when it comes to the illness at hand. Improving communication between doctors and patients would be an excellent investment for preventing diagnostic errors.

The other adage worth remembering is that the most important part of the stethoscope is the part between the earpieces. The work of Graber, Singh, and other researchers has demonstrated that most medical errors in diagnosis are cognitive, and so we have to pay attention to how we train clinicians to think, something I'll touch on more in chapter 14. In nearly every diagnostic situation, there's almost always a certain part of our stethoscopes that could stand to be tuned a little more finely.

# CHAPTER SIX

# THE DESCENT

Jay had been in the hospital since Saturday, when he'd spiked his first post-chemo fever. All through the weekend his fever raged, despite antibiotics. Over the course of Sunday, Tara grew increasingly worried about his difficulty breathing, although a chest X-ray didn't show a pneumonia or fluid in his lungs. He'd been continually complaining that his stomach felt full. In Tara's opinion, his abdomen seemed swollen, as did his feet. But the blood cultures had finally provided a definitive answer on Monday morning—MRSA. Methicillin-resistant staph aureus isn't a calming diagnosis by any stretch, but once you have a diagnosis, you can at least construct a plan of action. For Jay, the plan consisted of two things—an antibiotic specifically for MRSA and removal of his indwelling catheter, since catheters top the suspect list when bloodborne staph infections are diagnosed.

Because the recent chemotherapy had devastated all his cell lines, he didn't possess sufficient platelets to protect him from internal hemorrhage upon removal of the catheter, so Jay had to wait for hours as unit after unit of platelets were transfused into his veins. By 5 p.m., the platelet count was finally high enough, and the catheter was removed in the operating room. Afterward, Jay added another post to his blog: "Just got back from having my line out. Since this was the source of the infection, I should begin to fight it out and begin to recover. They may put another line in—by the end of the week is a possibility. Thanks for everyone's support. It has meant the world to me. Everyone's been so very helpful. Jay."

But even those few lines were a struggle to write. Every effort, it seemed, tired him out. Even speaking was exhausting, and Jay was reduced to whispers for the entire day. Using the urinal was a Herculean task that consumed every ounce of breath. At 8 p.m., Dr. Amir came by. Jay mustered his strength to force out three agitated words: "I . . . can't . . . breathe."

"Jay seems really anxious," Dr. Amir said to Tara. "We can give him something to help him relax." He ordered some Ativan for sedation and Ambien for sleep.

"What about all the Tylenol he's getting round the clock for his fevers?" Tara asked. "That could be affecting his liver, and that's where he's complaining of pain."

Dr. Amir didn't think the Tylenol was causing the pain. "His liver enzymes are only a little bit elevated, not enough to be toxicity from Tylenol. Besides, he needs the Tylenol because of his fevers."

Jay continued to have chills throughout the evening and required additional Demerol to control them. He kept pointing to his abdomen and saying it hurt. Tara finally hunted down the nurse to get him something stronger for the pain. Tara had to work in the ER the following morning, so she tried to get some rest that night. But it was nearly impossible. The spasms of worry, along with the rasps of Jay's breathing, rattled her sleep.

The predawn hours in a hospital offer up a spectral stillness, a foreboding semidarkness that is a breeding ground for apprehension and doubt. Tara tried in vain to still her agitated thoughts. Was she overreacting to insignificant things? It was hard for her to tell. Or was the staff blithely ignoring concerning clinical signs? In the bewildering limbo that she and Jay now inhabited, it was impossible to know which way was up.

Tara considered herself a reasonably experienced nurse, having worked in critical-care units in addition to her years in the ER. But she wasn't an oncology nurse. She hadn't spent extensive time with cancer patients and wasn't versed in the highly specialized care of bone marrow transplant units. She didn't presume to know the intricacies of chemotherapy agents or bone marrow transplantation. That was legitimately beyond her expertise.

But still . . .

It was 5 a.m. when Tara was roused by Jay's struggling to breathe. His heart was racing and his temperature was 103. "There's a puppy on top of the TV," Jay whispered hoarsely. "People are laundering money here."

Tara called the night nurse. "Jay is hallucinating," she reported.

"It's probably from the sleeping pills that he received," the nurse replied.

Sedatives can definitely cause hallucinations, as can the very act of being hospitalized. Disorientation, fevers, dehydration, and interrupted sleep/wake cycles can all cause hallucinations in hospitalized patients.

But still . . .

When Tara emptied his urinal, she saw that his urine—what little there was—shone a dark amber, the color of heavy oak. She noticed that his toenails were pale blue and his hands were puffy. His breathing was ragged.

It was early Tuesday morning already, though still technically the night shift by the hospital clock. Tara convinced the nurse to wake up Dr. Amir—the overnight doctor—because of Jay's labored breathing. Dr. Amir drew a blood gas from one of Jay's arteries to measure the level of oxygen. (Standard blood tests are drawn from veins, but venous blood does not reflect the true level of oxygen that the body's organs are receiving; arterial blood is needed for this.) The results showed that Jay was hypoxic, that his oxygen level was critically low. "He probably has ARDS," Dr. Amir said, before he left the hospital that morning. "He'll probably get moved to the ICU later today."

ARDS—acute respiratory distress syndrome—isn't a disease, per se. It's an acute inflammation of the air sacs of the lungs that can be precipitated by a host of conditions including severe pneumonia, sepsis, burns, drug reactions, and pancreatitis. The air sacs—the alveoli—are physiologic tollbooths that allow the oxygen breathed into the lungs to be transferred into the blood, which then fans out to supply the organs of the entire body. When the alveoli are inflamed, you can pump in all the oxygen you want, but the blood can't effectively receive it.

ARDS—if that was what Jay had—is an ICU-level emergency. There is no specific treatment, but patients need aggressive medical care while whatever caused the ARDS is treated. Most patients require intubation so that a ventilator can take over the work of breathing. However, this is not a panacea because pushing air in from a machine doesn't solve the issue of inflamed and recalcitrant alveoli.

Dr. Amir had said that Jay would likely go to the ICU, but as a fellow—and a covering, overnight fellow, at that—he didn't have any say in the overall direction of Jay's care. Besides, he was already gone. Tara called her boss in the ER and said she wouldn't be able to do her shift that day.

Jay received a stronger oxygen mask that helped increase his oxygen levels somewhat. It was hard to take an oral temperature because of the jagged breathing, but in his underarm, the thermometer read 104. When the day nurse did her morning rounds, Tara pointed out that Jay's lips and toes seemed bluish. The nurse pressed some buttons on the IV pump, jotted a few things on the paper she was holding, but didn't make eye contact with Tara. "It was as if the staff were pulling away from us," Tara told me.

Tara accompanied Jay for an early-morning CT scan of his chest, since yesterday's X-ray hadn't provided any answers. A CT could help determine whether there was a pneumonia, or an abscess, or maybe a blood clot, any of which could cause ARDS. After they arrived in the CT suite, Jay's bed was wheeled into the scanner and Tara was left in the deserted waiting area. She suddenly felt so alone, so utterly lost. Jay was spiraling down in front of her eyes and nothing she could do or say could stem this. It felt as though she were speaking a foreign language and no one on the staff could understand her. Was she going crazy? Had reality abandoned her?

The sweltering grimness of the waiting room hung heavy, siphoning off any traces of hope. For the first time since Jay was diagnosed, Tara felt her nursing fortitude begin to falter. Her skills and knowledge were failing her, and she could not seem to help him. It was all so insurmountable. She wilted into the armrest of the worn leatherette seat, sobbing uncontrollably for the duration of the CT scan.

Dr. Mueller, the hematology attending, came to Jay's room around 10 a.m. with the results of the CT scan. It showed a pneumonia at the base of Jay's right lung, plus fluid around the lungs (pleural effusions) on both sides. Also, his liver was enlarged. She would consult the pulmonary service about the pneumonia and pleural effusions. Tara had regrouped somewhat since breaking down in the CT suite. "Will you also be consulting GI about the enlarged liver and ongoing abdominal pain?" she asked.

Dr. Mueller demurred, saying that it would be up to the pulmonologist. "What about the ARDS?" Tara pressed. "Is Jay going to the ICU?"

"That will be the pulmonologist's decision," Dr. Mueller replied. There was a flat tone to her voice, almost curt. For Tara it felt like a blunt message: stop asking so many questions, stop making our work more difficult, stay out of Jay's care.

It was two agonizing hours until the pulmonologist arrived, but it may as well have been two hundred. Everything seemed to be riding on this doctor. Tara was on edge, ready to erupt, but at the same time utterly depleted, hardly able to maintain a cogent thought in her sleep-deprived state. The pulmonologist, Dr. Peterson, arrived shortly after Jay had received a dose of morphine. Tall, thin, and balding, Dr. Peterson parked himself at the foot of the bed. "So, what's going on?" he said.

Jay was unable to speak loudly enough or clearly enough to make himself understood. He looked to Tara with exhausted eyes. Tara turned to the pulmonologist. "Jay has been dyspneic and tachypneic since yesterday morning," she said.

"Those are fancy words," Dr. Peterson said. The snide tone was unmistakable. He rocked back on his heels, hands jammed into the front pockets of his white coat, mostly making eye contact with the linoleum floor. "Where'd you learn those?"

Tara didn't want to start a turf battle or raise anyone's hackles. Her goal was to help Jay, not prove any point. She replied calmly but cautiously, "I'm an

ER nurse, and I have some critical-care experience. I'm concerned about Jay's increased work of breathing, the swelling in his feet and hands, and especially his distended abdomen, which is making it hard for him to breathe. I am hoping that you'll move him to the ICU and maybe intubate him."

Dr. Peterson did not lift his eyes from the linoleum or offer any reaction. ("He acted as if I'd just read him a segment from the phone book," Tara recalled.) He moved around to the side of the bed to listen to Jay's lungs. He had Jay sit up, which Jay did lethargically, and listened at the back. "His lungs sound clear," Dr. Peterson announced, straightening up. "This is not a primary respiratory problem. I looked at the CT scan—there's no pneumonia."

For Tara, this was bordering on surreal. Yes, she was surviving on hardly any sleep and hadn't eaten more than a few bites in days, but earlier in the morning Dr. Mueller had said there were crackles in Jay's lungs. And later in the morning she said the CT scan showed pneumonia. Had Tara misheard? Or misunderstood?

"With my twenty-plus years' experience," Dr. Peterson continued, mainly toward the floor, "I can tell you that Jay doesn't have pneumonia or fluid inside his lungs. His lungs are being constricted by the pleural effusions—the fluid *around* the lungs. This is simply atelectasis." Atelectasis is a small, usually benign collapse of the lower parts of the lung. Most patients after surgery, for example, experience some atelectasis because they haven't been breathing as deeply as normal.

"But what about his work of breathing?" Tara persisted, gesturing toward Jay.

"Looks like morphine's doing the trick," Dr. Peterson said. It was hard for Tara to tell if this was pure sarcasm or straight-up condescension. The slight chuckle in his tone made her think the latter. Was it because she was a nurse that he was talking down to her? Was it because she was a woman? Was it because she barely reached five-foot-three even with her sturdiest nursing clogs on? Or was he like this to everyone?

Morphine has been used for eons to relieve shortness of breath. In palliative-care situations it can be a godsend. In acute situations, morphine can be extremely effective, but it treats only the symptom of breathlessness, not the underlying cause.

Tara knew she could not afford to be intimidated or to take offense. Even from a condescending cad. She forced herself to respond as evenly as possible. "What about BiPAP?" she asked. "Can we try him on some BiPAP?" BiPAP is a special breathing mask that uses pressure to forcefully push oxygen into the lungs. It's less invasive than intubation, so it is often used as a temporizing measure for patients who need assistance with breathing.

Dr. Peterson shook his head dismissively. "If anything we need to *decrease* his oxygen so that we can accurately trend his oxygenation. Right now, his oxygen saturation reads 100%, so he's probably getting too much oxygen." Normal oxygen saturation is in the high 90s. Dr. Peterson leaned over the bed and turned down the nozzle on the oxygen a little bit.

"But what about his edema?" Tara asked. "His hands and legs are swollen."

The doctor's body language was as flat as his affect. "The edema is just cosmetic."

"Don't you think he's in fluid overload?" Tara asked incredulously. "He's net *in* by two liters, and his urinary output is down."

"If anything, he needs *more* fluids," Dr. Peterson said. Patients with fevers have a higher fluid requirement, and most patients post-chemotherapy require additional hydration. "I'd want the Lasix stopped, even though he has slight crackles."

*Wait*, thought Tara. *Wait! Didn't he just say before that Jay's lungs were clear? Now he says there are crackles?* It was all so disorienting. To Tara, Jay looked sick, worsening by the moment. But the nurses on the unit didn't seem to think so. The hematology attending didn't seem to think so. The pulmonologist—a critical-care specialist—didn't seem to think so. Was she misreading everything? It was like stumbling through a house of distorted mirrors.

As Tuesday afternoon wore on, Tara grew more and more distraught. Jay's chest, back, and neck were mottled bluish-gray. His hands were now as swollen as his feet, and he complained of an uncomfortable tingling sensation in his limbs. Now his right knee was hurting. When the nurse came to hang a bag of saline, Tara asked her about the coloration of Jay's skin. "It's a side effect of the chemo," she answered.

Tara knew that her knowledge base did not extend to the intricacies of oncology. But still, was *everything* a side effect of chemo? How could that possibly be? Jay kept pointing to the right side of his abdomen, that it was still hurting. It was hard for him to speak, but he was able to signal a six with his fingers when Tara asked him to rate his pain on a scale of one to ten.

Later in the afternoon on Tuesday, Tara finally got a meeting with Dr. Mueller and Constance,* the nurse manager of the floor. In the conference room, Tara told them how unhappy she was with the care Jay was get-

---

*I recognize that the practice of referring to nurses by their first names and doctors by their last names underscores an unfortunate legacy of hierarchy (and, frankly, sexism). I am using "Constance," though, because that's how Tara referred to her and also because it reflects the reality that nurses generally permit patients and families to call them by their first names.

ting. "He's been tachypneic since Monday morning and has had abdominal pain since Sunday night. No one can continue to breathe like that. I think he's going to crash."

When there was no response to her blunt assessment, Tara said, "I want Jay to be transferred to the ICU. Maybe he needs to be electively intubated."

Intubation—getting a breathing tube inserted in order to allow a ventilator to take over—often takes place during an emergency, such as when a patient has a cardiac arrest or goes into shock. In emergencies like these, intubation can be life-saving, though it's a very stressful, high-stakes situation (quite unlike the calm, controlled intubation that an anesthesiologist does before surgery).

*Elective* intubation is the decision to insert a breathing tube *before* a patient reaches an emergency situation. If you think the patient will ultimately need it, better to put it in before the chaos of blood pressure bottoming out or the heart or lungs ceasing to function. Of course you'd never want to electively intubate a patient who *didn't* need it, since this is quite an invasive procedure with many potential harms to the patient. It's a decision not to be taken lightly.

Dr. Mueller said, "We don't electively intubate here at this hospital." She glanced over at Constance, and Tara thought she caught a smile between the doctor and nurse. "We've dealt with this before," Dr. Mueller added. Tara looked at her quizzically. Did she mean they'd dealt with this sort of clinical situation before or they'd dealt with pesky family members from the medical profession before?

"A little bit of medical knowledge," Dr. Mueller went on, "can be a dangerous thing."

*So that's it,* Tara thought. *They are just sick of me bothering them. I'm just that annoying family member. I'm that bothersome nurse getting in their way. They want me to just disappear so they won't have to deal with me.*

Tara took a deep breath to steady herself. It had been eight and a half weeks since Jay first picked up that Hula Hoop. Eight and a half weeks of what seemed like a descent into an alternate universe, an incomprehensible netherworld that refused to right itself. "I understand that you have gone to school a lot longer than me," she said to Dr. Mueller, endeavoring to keep her emotions in check. "And I know that you know more than I do about oncology, but I still don't see how Jay can keep up this increased work of breathing that he's been doing for the past thirty hours."

Dr. Mueller's tone softened a bit. "Don't get me wrong, your husband is definitely sick. But"—and here she sounded firmer—"he's not sick enough. Maybe in a smaller hospital, he would be in the ICU, but not here."

*Is she being sarcastic?* Tara wondered. *Is it just the ego of a big-city hospital?* She felt like she might vomit, right there in the conference room, as she realized that no one, not one single person, was going to help her get Jay to an ICU. She considered trying to transfer Jay to another hospital, but he was clearly too sick for that. Tara racked her brain to come up with something, anything, to get help for Jay. Anything to get their attention. "Knee pain," she blurted out. "Jay's been complaining about right-knee pain for the last few hours." She knew that the knee pain was minor in the grand scheme of things, but she was desperate to get the medical team back to Jay's bedside. Knee pain in a patient with a bloodborne infection could indicate infection of the joint, so it was a symptom that the doctors would be obligated to investigate.

Dr. Mueller seemed willing to placate her in order to end the meeting. "I'll stop in and take a look at his knee before I leave for the day, okay?"

*No*, Tara thought, *no it's not okay*! But she realized it was all she was going to get. Tara could barely lift her feet to walk as she left the room. She had never felt so helpless—as a nurse or as a human being—as she did right now. No matter what she said or did for Jay, she could not make the great machinations of the hospital grind forward.

The social worker happened to be standing right there when Tara stepped into the hallway. "These people deal with this every day," she told Tara reassuringly. "Trust them." Tara could hear snippets of laughter drifting out from behind the door of the conference room she'd just left. Constance and Dr. Mueller were probably laughing about something else altogether—she'd certainly been on the other side of that divide—but she imagined they were laughing at her and her pitiful efforts to play doctor.

Tara waited nervously for Dr. Mueller to arrive to evaluate Jay's knee. Jay's skin tone was slate-gray now, and his respiratory rate was in the forties. The dark-blue mottling seemed to creep out from under his gown up toward his face. He was restless, complaining again of the tingling in his hands and feet. When the nurse came to take vital signs, Tara asked about it.

"It's a side effect of the chemo," the nurse answered. She jotted down the vitals and then left the room.

Jay's feet were swollen and ice-cold. Tara reached down to warm them, massaging them gently to coax in some heat. "Does that help?" she asked. She couldn't hear Jay's answer, so she leaned in closer to him.

"I love you," he whispered, and Tara began to shake with panic. From the corner of her eye she noticed blood oozing from Jay's chest, from where the indwelling catheter used to be. She grabbed the call button and pressed it desperately, even though she knew the nurses were sick of her.

It was nearly 4 p.m. when Dr. Mueller finally arrived, almost an hour after their conversation in the conference room. She made a beeline for Jay's right knee, bending it and palpating the joint. She shrugged, not seeming to find much there. Then she pulled back to look at the rest of him and it was almost as though she was seeing Jay for the first time. "How long has his skin been like that?" Dr. Mueller asked, slowly. Her voice was now hard-edged with concern.

"Since lunchtime," Tara answered curtly. "The nurse said it was a side effect of the chemo."

Dr. Mueller hardly waited for Tara to finish her sentence. The panic was visible in her eyes. "That is *not* normal," the hematologist said, rushing out of the room to order a stat blood gas.

Ten minutes passed, and Tara was still alone. She checked Jay's oxygen saturation on the monitor and it was 82%. She pressed the call button again. No one came. Tara dashed out to the hallway and saw Dr. Mueller on the phone in the nurses' station. The time for niceties was over. "Jay's saturation is down to 82%!" she bellowed at Dr. Mueller. "He's crashing."

"I've ordered a stat blood gas," Dr. Mueller replied, but her voice sounded uncharacteristically nervous.

Tara rushed back to Jay's room. "Where the hell is that stat blood gas," Tara barked hoarsely at the two nurses who'd finally arrived, but they didn't know. The nurses tried to get an oxygen saturation reading, but now the monitor wouldn't pick up anything. They tried it on Jay's fingers, on his toes, on his ears, on his forehead, but no reading. They tried another machine in case the first one wasn't working, and then another.

Tara watched them in disbelief. It was crystal clear to her that the nurses couldn't get a reading, not because the machines were faulty, but because Jay's entire vascular system was clamping down. "He has to be intubated," Tara shouted.

Jay pointed feebly to his bladder, indicating that he had to urinate. They brought the urinal to him and out came one hundred cc's of blood. Tara became frantic. "His kidneys are going," she screamed at the nurses. "He has to be moved to the ICU!"

Another fifteen minutes went by before the tech finally arrived to do the blood gas. Of course it was impossible to find Jay's pulse at this point so the tech couldn't get an arterial blood sample. It was 4:40 when Tara heard Dr. Mueller yell from the hallway, "Call a rapid response!"

"It's about damn time," Tara shouted back from Jay's room, shaking with panic and relief at the same time.

Rapid response teams developed in hospitals after the recognition that once a cardiac or pulmonary arrest has occurred, it is rare to get a meaningful "save," no matter how assiduous the code team is. The idea came about, then, to create an emergency team to intervene *before* the code occurs. You wouldn't have to wait until the patient actually lost their pulse or respiration (i.e., coded) to get intensive help—you could activate the assistance of an ICU-level team to the bedside as soon as the patient's clinical situation began to deteriorate. The goal was to prevent the code before it happened.

As soon as the rapid response was activated, a flood of people descended upon Jay's room. As they were gowning up, though, Jay began to gasp for air, gurgling and grunting. "God damn it," Tara exploded. "You people should have listened to me! Now he's agonal-breathing! He should have been intubated this morning!" As Jay's breathing withered away, the rapid response team switched into cardiac-arrest mode, sliding a board under Jay's back so they could begin CPR.

As Jay was rolled to the side to get the board under him, his head was briefly turned toward Tara. For a second, Tara and Jay were eye to eye and she watched as his pupils suddenly widened to the maximum possible. In medical terminology, he'd blown his pupils—an ominous sign of the brain swelling and beginning to push out of the skull into the vertebral column.

"You fuckers!" Tara screamed at everyone and at no one. "He's unresponsive now! I told all of you, but no one would listen! I told you he was getting worse all day!"

The code proceeded in the standard manner that codes do, the standard manner that was oh so familiar to Tara in her professional role but stutteringly otherworldly right now. At the head of the bed someone was intubating Jay and then squeezing an Ambu bag to press air through the tube into his lungs. Another team member was throwing his full bodyweight into CPR through his interlocked hands, lurching the bed with each compression. Someone else was jamming vials of epinephrine and atropine into the IVs to corral Jay's heart and vasculature into action. Another person was furiously drawing labs. A nurse stood in the corner, methodically charting the proceedings.

Tara spotted Dr. Mueller at the back of the room. The hematologist was looking up to the ceiling with her hands clasped in front of her, almost in a prayer pose. "You did this!" Tara hissed at her. "You're going to be sorry."

CPR was briefly halted to check the heart rhythm. "PEA," someone announced and Tara could feel the floor careering out from beneath her. Pulseless electrical activity is a perilous state in which the heart is firing electrical signals but these aren't translating into meaningful cardiac contractions that could ultimately be detected as a pulse. It's a sign of a desperately flailing heart. Tara ran out of the room screaming, not knowing which way to turn.

Constance confronted her in the hallway. "You can't make a scene like this, Tara." She pointed a finger at Tara's face, scolding her, nurse to nurse. "If you keep on like this, we'll have to have you removed."

"That's bullshit, Constance," Tara spat back. "I *told* everyone this was going to happen and you all ignored me." The two of them stood there, a foot apart. Through gritted teeth Tara said, "Go ahead and *try* to make me leave." She spun away from the nurse manager and returned to Jay's room.

The code was in full swing, simultaneously chaotic and controlled. Gowned, gloved, and masked bodies entombed the space around Jay's bed. Sweaty desperation hung heavy in the air. Tara's volcanic anger now began to leach away in the agitating churn of bodies, machines, protocols, hierarchy, and apprehension. Disbelief became numbness and she could feel herself almost slipping away.

In the middle of this, a nurse Tara had never seen before materialized in the room. She wordlessly guided Tara to a chair and coaxed her into it. The nurse kneeled in front of Tara and took her hand. "I'm an ER nurse also," she said. "Like you." She kept up a soft stream of words as Tara sat there, nearly catatonic.

"She had the presence of an angel," Tara recalled. "To this day, I am not even sure if she was real or just a figment of my imagination."

"We have a pulse," someone shouted, and Tara felt the dubious arrow of hope stab into her. Jay's heart was now beating! A surgical team had arrived to insert a central venous line, since Jay had only two small IVs after the indwelling catheter had been removed and they were insufficient for the massive resuscitation efforts. The surgeons and the code team debated whether to insert the line right there in the room or to move Jay to an OR where the environment was sterile. They decided that the OR would be better, now that Jay had a pulse, and began the preparations to transport him.

They hadn't made it out of the room when Jay's rhythm and pulse were lost again. Someone jumped on the bed to resume CPR. The code began again in earnest.

For Tara, the scene was both unfathomably intimate and piercingly brutal. It was as if a serrated grater was rasping away at her, flaying deeper through skin, muscle, and bone. At the same time, though, she was entirely numb. How was it possible to simultaneously be in so much pain but also feel nothing? Time was spooling both backward and forward. The code was going on forever—round after round of epinephrine, atropine, CPR—but was also unimaginably fleeting.

The ER nurse who'd been sitting with Tara looked her in the eye for what seemed like forever. "Tara," she said quietly, "you might need to make a decision here."

Tara knew what she meant. She had been on that nurse's side of the conversation many times before. She'd been the one to ask the distraught family members when to stop the resuscitation efforts. She'd been the one to present what seemed like a life-or-death decision but really wasn't. It was a death-or-death decision, the two options separated only by an arbitrary sliver of time.

Tara gathered the last remnants of her clinical reserve and asked two questions: "How long has he been down? What's his rhythm been?"

The answers came: "Forty minutes." "PEA."

She didn't have to look at Jay to know, but she did nevertheless. He was blue. His skin was mottled and leathery. He was dead.

"Call the code," she whispered to them, hospital shorthand for ending resuscitation.

And like all nurses do, she instinctively noted the time. It was 5:20 p.m.

# CHAPTER SEVEN

# FOR THE RECORD

I have participated in scores of codes like Jay's. Mostly, like Jay's, they were not successful. Nearly every patient who codes dies because of the simple tautology that it is crushing illness that brings them to the doorstep of the code. In a strange way, death is actually one of the steps of the code. It isn't listed in the algorithm, of course, but it's there. The first step. Everyone knows it, but no one will say it. Even though the patient has already died from the devastation of disease, the code presses on until someone "calls it." Then, and only then, can death be acknowledged. It is a wrenching combination of human grief and quotidian bureaucracy.

As a resident, I was always struck by the odd concept of "time of death," especially when I become the one in charge of the code. On the one hand, I would announce it with scientific precision ("4:17 a.m."). On the other hand, it was entirely arbitrary. If I'd decided to continue the code for another minute, the time of death would be 4:18 a.m. If I'd faced up to reality a bit sooner, the time of death might be 4:14 a.m. In all cases, life had already ceased for the patient. In fact, life had ceased before the code started. *That* was the time when the patient had stopped breathing or the heart had stopped beating. *That* was when the patient had really died. Yet we officially record the time of death as the moment when we adjourn *our* battle, not the moment the cells have adjourned theirs.

I suspect this relates to the way the medical record dominates healthcare. Everything that transpires during the course of a patient's contact with the healthcare system must—for good reason—be documented. The chart (also called the medical record) is the chronical of a patient's medical odyssey. Every medication given, every lab test, every X-ray is part of the chart. Doctors and nurses write progress notes, documenting the patient's current condition and the plan of care. Even during the chaos of a code, there will always be one nurse who stands calmly in the corner, fastidiously documenting each incremental step of the resuscitation effort. The final entry in that running document, of course, is the time of death.

To me, this reflects how the medical chart often ends up dictating medical practice, rather than the reverse. As documentation demands grow, our practices change in order to accommodate. For generations, the medical record consisted of the standard paper chart, with various team members scribbling their observations in one unified physical location. The chronical was an actual chronical you could leaf through to read the patient's entire story. Of course, you could also accidentally spill your coffee on that lofty chronical. Or your Thai red curry. The chart could get knocked to the floor—52 pickup–style— by an orderly bustling by and end up with its pages hopelessly out of order. It could be buried under a pile of journals on the desk of an endocrinologist who left for a week's vacation. The discharge summary could have been written by a surgeon with Neolithic penmanship skills. Three key pages could have been "borrowed" by a medical student for a 7 a.m. conference.

So there are a host of compelling reasons for the medical chart to be digitized. The electronic medical record, known as the EMR (sometimes called the EHR, for electronic health record), obviates most of those shortcomings—it's always legible and it can't be stranded in someone's office. If you spill your coffee *and* your Thai red curry on it, you might short-circuit your computer terminal, but the actual EMR will survive.

The EMR may be less tangible than the old paper chart, but if anything it exerts an even stronger influence over how medical care is delivered. For reasons both intentional and unintentional, the EMR has fundamentally changed how health professionals process medical information. In the paper-chart days, each time I saw a patient, I was given a blank piece of paper—a blank tableau, you might say. (In Bellevue, for some inexplicable reason, the progress-note paper was flamingo pink. For my entire medical training I felt as though I were floundering in a sea of Pepto-Bismol.)

The beauty of the blank sheet of paper was that I could write down my thoughts in exactly the order in which I processed them. I would start with the patient's main reason for the visit ("the Chief Complaint") and the HPI ("History of Present Illness), and then follow with the past medical history. After I examined the patient, I would note the physical exam findings, followed by the pertinent lab or radiology results.

Here I'd stop and think, trying to pull it together. I'd run through my differential diagnosis. If I wasn't overly rushed, I'd flesh out a detailed assessment, explicating my clinical reasoning as to why I might favor one diagnosis over another. Lastly, I'd pen my explicit plan of action. My goal was that I—or anyone else—could come back to this note at some later time and immediately grasp the entirety of what I was thinking and understand *why* I was thinking it.

In contrast, when I open up the EMR, the computer forces me to document in *its* order, which has no relationship to the arc of my thoughts. This reflects the fact that EMRs were initially developed as billing systems. Only later did they start to incorporate clinical information, and even the best of the EMRs do not think the way clinicians think. We humans must be rerouted to the EMR's requirements.

Not only does the EMR interfere with the train of thought, it also forces its users to compartmentalize their thinking. Each aspect of the patient is contained in a different field, and these fields aren't logically connected. On the old paper note, I could group the blood test results and the X-ray results together because they logically formed supporting data to prove or disprove a diagnosis. I could jot down the upshot of a cardiology consultation within my assessment, if the result was relevant to my clinical reasoning. But in the EMR, the lab results are in one place, and the radiology results in another, and the consultations are in a third place.

This fragmentation of thinking is particularly dangerous when it comes to diagnosis, a process that, as we've seen, requires *integration* of information. The EMR conspires against integration by forcing information, as well as your flow of thought, into a rigid structure that is convenient for computer programmers and the billing department but not necessarily logical for anyone taking care of patients.

There's no going back from the EMR, and I don't think we *should* go back. The advantages of centralized medical information are substantial. But the consequences of the EMR—however unintended they may be—are equally substantial and have potent ramifications for medical care as well as medical error.

---

Robert Wachter, an internist from the University of California-San Francisco, has written extensively about medicine and technology. Although an admitted techno-optimist, Wachter writes evenhandedly about the advances and the drawbacks of medical technology in his book *The Digital Doctor*.[1] The case that prompted him to write the book raises the hairs on the neck of any doctor, nurse, or patient who has ever been party to an EMR.

On a balmy July day, a pediatrics resident ordered Bactrim for a teenage patient named Pablo Garcia hospitalized in the wards of UCSF's Children's Hospital. Bactrim is one of those antibiotics that has been around for so long that no one even remembers what the milligram dosing is. The prescription is always "one tab, twice daily"—though with lower doses for patients with renal insufficiency and for young children. (Bactrim is actually a combination of two antibiotics—160 milligrams of trimethoprim and 800 milligrams of sulfamethoxazole.)

Pablo's weight was three pounds under the cutoff for the standard adult dosing (one tab, twice daily) so the EMR sent the resident down the pediatric pathway for weight-based dosing—5 milligrams per kilogram. Weight-based dosing is obviously critical in pediatrics, since children can range in size from 6 pounds to 85 pounds.

The weight calculation in this case led to a dose of 193 milligrams of trimethoprim, which is a bit larger than the tablet size of 160 milligrams. The resident correctly rounded down to the 160-milligram tablet. Such a rounding, though, triggers an automatic alert in the EMR to a pharmacist to double-check the dosing.

The pharmacist contacted the resident to clarify that 160 milligrams was the dose she indeed wanted. This was the EMR's way of trying to catch calculation errors—having a human intervene to double-check. The resident confirmed the dose with pharmacist and then reentered "160."

You can enter the dose of Bactrim in the EMR either by the standard milligram dosing (160 mg is one tab) or by weight-based dosing (milligrams per kilogram). Unfortunately, the EMR "defaulted" to the mg/kg unit that the resident had been using earlier. So instead of entering 160 *mg*, she inadvertently entered 160 *mg per kg*. That's 160 milligrams for every one of Pablo Garcia's thirty-eight kilograms.

You don't need to do the math to feel faint, but Wachter does it for us. The dose comes to 6,160 milligrams, or 38½ tabs of Bactrim.

Nearly every medical professional with a detectable pulse knows that Bactrim is a "one tab, twice daily" medication. We know it in the same way we know that the normal number of fingers on each hand is five. We would be as likely to dump 38½ packets of sugar in our morning coffee as to prescribe 38½ tabs of Bactrim. But once the error was embedded in the EMR, it took on a bizarrely vigorous life of its own. It was like watching the lead-up to a horror movie climax in excruciating slow motion. I found it almost unbearable to turn the pages.

The Bactrim order was now routed to the medication supply room. To avoid medical error the hospital had installed a state-of-the-art pharmacy robot. This machine could make none of the errors that humans might make—miscounting, misreading, yawning. As the order had already been labeled as "approved" by the human pharmacist, the robot duly dispensed 38½ tablets into the medication bin with 100% accuracy.

The nurse who received the medication bin on the ward was taken aback because she recognized that this was a very unusual number of pills. But she could see that the order had been double-checked by both doctor and pharmacist. This was reassuring. Plus, the bar-coding system that matched the pills to the patient (to prevent medication mix-up errors) assured her that this was the right dose for the right patient. And working in an academic medical center that handled more than its share of oddball diseases and experimental treatments, it wasn't unusual to see atypical dosing schedules.

If the nurse stopped her rounds to ask another nurse for advice or to page the doctor about the medication, an ominous red alert would pop up on her screen informing her—and her supervisor—that she was late in administering the meds. (Delivering medications on time is one of the many "quality measures" that hospitals emphasize.) Additionally, the EMR wouldn't allow an unsure nurse to decide, "I'll finish with my other patients first and then get back to this one when I can give it some extra thought," because her current task wouldn't be marked "complete" until she'd scanned and administered all 38½ pills to her patient. So there was no way to get help unless she pushed back against every disincentive and ground the whole ward to a halt. Not an easy thing to do on a busy ward under pressure to "be efficient."

And so, backed up by the assurance of the bar codes, the precision of the pharmacy robot, the documentation of human rechecking by both pharmacist and doctor—all measures instituted to decrease medical error—the nurse doled out the pills as instructed by the EMR. Thirty-eight horse-pill-size tablets of Bactrim. And, of course, that extra half tab.

At first Pablo noticed only some odd numbness and tingling. Then he became anxious and a little confused. Then suddenly his body erupted into full-blown seizures. He stopped breathing and a code was called. Pablo Garcia survived, miraculously, and apparently without permanent damage. But he easily could have ended up on dialysis or with permanent brain damage or dead. (It seemed like the dosage of *luck* on that day was quite a bit higher than normal—maybe even 38½ times higher.) He recovered, seemingly fully, though no doubt his trust in the medical system suffered permanent damage.

The case is so rattling because it highlights how an EMR that is trying to improve patient safety through its various alerts and warnings can instead end up harming a patient gravely. It's all the more ironic because this is an error that would have been caught in a flash if the doctor had written the order by hand instead of computer or if the medication had been dispensed by a pharmacist instead of a robot. The very technology we are counting on to decrease our medical-error rate can actually increase it, or create new kinds of errors.

Wachter uses this case to highlight, among other things, the issue of alerts, the basic tool the EMR brings to the table when it comes to preventing medical errors. For doctors and nurses, these computerized alerts constitute one continuous, communal migraine. Handling prescriptions and medication orders is what we do all day, and the alert system has become an octopus of misery, swatting unceasingly from all directions. Just when you think you may have cleared the gauntlet of alerts, another seven bulbous legs come whipping at you with more alerts to navigate.

Now, perhaps you think I'm being histrionic here, but that is certainly what it feels like. Every time I have to certify that a vitamin D pill is *not* a controlled substance, I want to scream. Every time I have to tend to the alert that warns me that drug interactions are "not available" for the walker I'm prescribing, I want to take a scalpel to the screen. When the alert informing me that a medication should be "prescribed with caution" for someone over sixty-five pops up for *every single medication* for *every single patient over sixty-five*, I'm ready to dismember the keyboard.

I'm angrier still because I know that buried within these useless alerts are some important ones. I *want* to be reminded if a medication is contraindicated in liver disease or needs to be dosed differently because of impaired renal function. I know that I can't possibly remember all the crucial drug interactions, so I want the EMR to catch me when I inadvertently prescribe two meds that can't go together. Thus I'm furious at the EMR for inundating me with so many banal alerts that I—like most doctors and nurses who are honest enough to admit it—end up ignoring them all.

After reading about the Bactrim disaster in Bob Wachter's book, I decided to rouse myself from complacency. After all, when the doctor ordered 38½ times the normal dose of Bactrim, the EMR *did* pop an alert in her face. But she had just finished reviewing the order with the pharmacist, so she dismissed the alert like she and I and everyone else do with the hundreds of alerts every hour that seem designed to prevent us from getting any work done.

I therefore committed myself to reading all the alerts before I dismissed them. There might be a crucial one buried in there, and I didn't want to miss it. Besides, the EMR is a legal document. Clicking "okay" to an alert indicates that I've read it, evaluated its contents, considered its impact, and then made a decision. That's certainly what a lawyer would say in court.

I set to work the very next morning, feeling like a boxer newly motivated in the ring, bobbing confidently, flexing my newly invigorated patient-safety muscles. I could almost feel the satiny robe glittering around my shoulders instead of my saggy white coat with ink stains from a leaky pen. I was ready for battle!

Let's just say I didn't even make it through the first round. I was defeated with my very first patient of the day. He needed thirteen prescriptions and there were several alerts for each medication, which added up to dozens of alerts. Nearly all were useless. Things like "weight-based dosing not available for this medication"—for a medication that does not need to be adjusted for weight. Or something equally unhelpful, like "drug interactions not available for this medication" when I'm prescribing alcohol swabs. Occasionally I'd get something of possible importance but couched in murkiness, such as "Drug X may increase bio-availability of drug Y. Quality of data uncertain." What was I supposed to do with that?

When I prescribed him a blood pressure cuff to check his pressure at home, that prescription set off a host of alerts. How could an eight-inch piece of vinyl interact with seven different medications? And, naturally, weight-based dosing was not available. My patient also committed the cardinal sin of being over sixty-five, so every single prescription—even his blood pressure cuff—was accompanied with the warning that I needed to "prescribe with caution."

But I persevered, reading and registering every single medication alert, no matter how inane. What ultimately felled me, what pushed me over the ropes completely, was that this patient was taking warfarin. Warfarin is an anti-coagulant, a so-called blood thinner, which he was taking because his atrial fibrillation put him at risk for blood clots and thus strokes.

Warfarin notoriously interacts with nearly every food, drug, and chemical in the universe, so the number of alerts it generates is distinctly epic. But warfarin is even more arduous because it's dosed according to its level in the blood, which changes constantly based on whether the patient overindulged in spinach, or took allergy pills after visiting a friend with a cat, or forgot to take cholesterol meds for a few days, or glanced more skeptically at Mars. The ongoing tinkering with warfarin dosing has a Rube Goldberg feel to it, and patients often end up on elaborate dosing combinations that change monthly, sometimes weekly.

Prescriptions for warfarin have to be rewritten more frequently than those for any other medication, and have the most intricate dosing combinations and the most drug interactions. The stakes are also much higher than with nearly any other medication, because if the dose is a smidge too low, you can cause clots and strokes. If the dose is a smidge too high, you can cause hemorrhage. Erring in either direction can severely harm or even kill a patient. You can see why warfarin is easily the most dreaded medication to prescribe.

My patient was on a not-atypical schedule of 8 milligrams on Tuesdays, Thursdays, Fridays, and Sundays, but 9 milligrams on Mondays, Wednesdays, and Saturdays. Warfarin does not come in 8- or 9-milligrams tabs, so I had to rely on the 4- and 5-milligram tablets and write separate prescriptions for each, plus a footnoted dissertation explaining how to take the pills correctly.

I had to limber up on advanced polynomials just to calculate how many tablets of what size on which day would be needed and how many of each added up to a one-month supply. And that was *before* facing the forty-six individual alerts that *each* of warfarin prescriptions elicited. (I believe I hold the Bellevue Hospital record with a set of warfarin prescriptions that elicited 241 individual alerts for an elderly patient who was taking a warehouse of interacting medications. I eventually dug out my old prescription pad and wrote the prescriptions by hand. It took seven seconds.)

Suffice it to say that my adventure in reading every single medication alert didn't improve the quality of the medical care for this patient. In fact, it didn't leave any *room* for medical care, since it consumed just about the entire visit. As his physician, I certainly didn't gain anything from the process other than an ulcer and a waiting room full of annoyed patients whose appointments were delayed. I threw a skeptical look at Mars and then spent the rest of the day doing what most doctors do—blindly clicking "okay" to alerts that bloom by the dozens, not reading a single one, hoping and praying that we're not missing something that really counts.

What burns my colleagues and me the most, though, is the motivation behind these alerts. It's so clear to us that the first priority is attending to liability rather than to patient care. If they've posted every possible warning, no matter how lame, then they—the hospital, the EMR, the greater universe—cannot be held at fault if something goes wrong. It's the doctor who clicked "okay" to the warnings who is at fault.

The whole warning system feels like a transfer of blame—not to mention workload—onto the medical staff. Doctors and nurses, of course, have no other option but to plug through the sea of alerts because we have to get the medications to our patients. It's estimated that primary care doctors spend a full hour per day just responding to alerts.[2] While EMRs have decreased[3] classic medication errors (by having standardized dosing and eliminating the penmanship problem), it is not clear that overall *harm* to patients has decreased, since new kinds of errors can be introduced, as we are seeing.

Wachter broadens the issue of alert fatigue from the EMR to all the alarms and bells that go off in the hospital, all of which exist to prevent medical error. In the five ICUs of his own hospital (which care for about sixty-six patients, on average) there are more than 2.5 million alarms each month—bells and beeps from all the monitors affixed to the patients. The vast majority of these are false alarms,[4] which leads the nurses and doctors to reflexively discount and silence most of them.

It was just such discounting and silencing that led to the cardiac arrest and death of a patient at Massachusetts General Hospital.[5] An elderly patient was in the cardiac unit because he needed a pacemaker. After eating breakfast on a January morning in 2010, he chatted with his visiting family. He then took a walk around the hospital floor and returned to his room. At 9:53 a.m., his heart rate began to slow. An alarm went off, but apparently none of the ten nurses on duty noticed it, or if they did, it didn't register as anything urgent. At some point, the alarm was manually silenced by a staff member. This could have been accidental, or it could have been that someone felt it was a false alarm. In either case, the alarm was disabled. So when the patient's heart rate continued its descent, there was no further alarm. When the heart rate hit zero, there was no sound at all. Not from the patient and not from any of the million-dollar technology affixed to his body. At 10:16 a.m., a nurse entered the room for a routine task and found the patient dead.

The *Boston Globe* issued a scathing investigative report that uncovered more than two hundred deaths over five years related to alarm fatigue. It found that nurses were bombarded with alarms, the vast majority of which were false. It didn't seem as though there was an epidemic of ineptitude among the nurses. Rather, there were just so many alarms that they were losing the ability to alarm anyone. They were simply background noise.

The stated goal of these alarms, like the medication alerts in the EMR, is to enhance patient safety, but, as this investigation highlighted, they can inadvertently cause harm. The alarms are designed to cast the net as widely as possible, because even one bad outcome could incur liability costs in the hundreds of millions of dollars to the manufacturers of these devices, the hospitals, and the EMRs. It is therefore in their interest to have the alarms go off at the slightest hint of abnormality. That the nurses are stuck in a hive of alarms is less of a concern to them.

What the EMRs and medical devices do *not* do is think the way nurses and doctors think.

Doctors and nurses are always prioritizing incoming signals. We can't possibly treat every signal as a critical emergency, so we relegate certain ones to the top of our concern and others to the bottom. Our EMR does try to color-code the alerts according to severity, but the middle level is still so voluminous that this doesn't do much to lessen the jungle of alerts that a doctor must traverse to complete a medication order. Alarms on cardiac monitors try to do the same thing, with differing pitches and frequency, but it hardly makes a dent in the sonic jungle that the average cardiac nurse has to function in.

Getting machines and EMRs to think a bit more like humans (while still retaining the encyclopedic, fatigueless abilities that humans lack) is clearly the goal. The various alerts and alarms would have to work together in a physiologic manner. For example, if a cardiac monitor shows no pulse, this typically sets off a code-red type of alarm. But in a smarter world, that alarm wouldn't go off if the blood pressure monitor is still recording a healthy blood pressure. (If your heart *truly* stops beating, you quickly lose any semblance of blood pressure.) "No pulse" would therefore be interpreted as the cardiac monitor being dislodged rather than the patient being close to death. A low-level alert could go to the nurse that the machinery needs to be adjusted. In this smarter world that Wachter imagines, alarms would be activated only if the various bits of data made clinical sense.

Similarly, the EMR could stand to acquire some clinical common sense that would adapt its alert system in a more logical way. For example, if a patient who's older than 65 has been taking lisinopril for 12 years there's no utility in sending a "prescribe with caution" alert because the patient has clearly tolerated the medication for longer than half the staff has been in practice. The EMR ought to be able to synthesize the warnings with a semblance of clinical relevance (and flush away the 50% that are utter fluff).

Wachter seems confident that this is possible, though it would require a major refocusing by the manufacturers. They'd have to spend far more time in the trenches with the medical staff to see how their products play out in the real world and to acquire a more realistic understanding of how medicine is practiced. They'd also have to work together to make their products compatible—something that might require putting patient safety above profits.

I can't put all the blame on the manufacturers—although it would feel intensely satisfying for ten solidly self-righteous minutes—because they didn't create the litigious environment that we all inhabit, something I'll discuss later in the book. Manufacturers very reasonably want to do everything to avoid lawsuits, even if it ends up depositing more work and additional misery on doctors and nurses.

The litigious environment, however, is one of the ways that EMR-related errors come to light. A survey of malpractice cases demonstrated the variety (and severity) of harms that can befall patients due to the EMR. Mark Graber and his colleagues analyzed 248 malpractice cases in which the EMR was somehow implicated, either because of the system itself or how a staff member used the system.[6] An example of a systems-related error was a "chief complaint" field that accepted only a limited number of characters. In this case, the patient had complained of "sudden onset of chest pains with burning epigastric pain, some relief with antacid." Because of the field-size limitations, the chief complaint came through only as "epigastric pain." No one did an EKG, and the patient suffered a major cardiac event a few days later.

An example of a user-related error was a case where somebody copied and pasted a previous note. The previous note had neglected to mention that the patient was taking the potent anti-arrhythmic drug amiodarone. That oversight was thus repeated in the current note. The patient—who needed the medication for his arrhythmia—was then given a new prescription for amiodarone and ended up getting double the dose and experienced toxic side effects.

A number of cases centered on delayed or missed diagnoses, especially of cancer but also of many other serious illnesses. In some cases there was a delay in getting results of tests into the computer system or the test results didn't get routed to the right person. In other cases the results were sitting in the doctor's queue and simply hadn't been noticed.

Much of this comes down to basic usability. Even if an EMR is perfectly designed to avoid error, it won't succeed if it's so clunky to use that nurses end up improvising shortcuts just to survive the day. Even if the system appropriately alerts doctors to every possible drug interaction, it won't succeed if the doctors feel drowned by the blizzard of alerts and blindly okay them all just to get a prescription done.

Although these EMR-related cases were only a small fraction of the total number of malpractice cases, they highlight the unique vulnerability that exists at the nexus of humans and technology. Minor flaws in technology can cross-pollinate with minor human flaws, with the potential to multiply to a devastating end.

On September 20, 2014, Thomas Eric Duncan flew to Dallas, Texas, from his home in Monrovia, Liberia. Three days later he started to feel rotten—his stomach hurt, he was nauseated, he felt feverish. The next night, on September 25, he went to the ER of Texas Health Presbyterian Hospital. On any given day hundreds of people show up in ERs with symptoms that sound like a stomach flu. But this wasn't any given day. West Africa was in the throes of an Ebola outbreak that would ultimately infect almost 30,000 (and kill more than 11,000) in the three countries most affected: Guinea, Sierra Leone, and Liberia.[7]

The rest of the world was bracing for the Ebola epidemic to spread internationally, given how easily the disease was spread person to person. Hospitals were ramping up their protocols to crisis levels. Bellevue Hospital, where I work, serves a diverse and well-traveled clientele, so we were racing at full speed to prepare. Everyone from the clerical staff to the upper administrative echelons was drilled to be on the lookout for two key factors: recent travel to the endemic area and presence of a fever. The immediate first step was to isolate the patient. (Our medical clinic had to designate one room to be the Ebola isolation room, and my office—being closest to the entrance—drew the short straw. The stacks of literary journals on my file cabinet had to go, replaced by masks, gowns, and gloves, plus folders full of emergency response plans. Maintenance workers sawed a hole in my door to create a glass window so that healthcare workers could communicate with potentially infected patients from a distance, without risking close contact. Post-Ebola, my literary journals have regained their spot, but I still have the window, which now has to be covered with sheets of copy paper to protect patient privacy.)

Thomas Eric Duncan had both red-alert signs: a fever and recent travel from Liberia. Yet he was sent home, along with a prescription for antibiotics. The nurse, in her triage note, indicated that the patient had recently been in West Africa. But the doctor didn't see the nurse's note, so the fever and the travel history weren't connected. Consideration of Ebola therefore did not enter his diagnostic thought process.

Forty-eight hours later, on September 28, Duncan called 911 and was brought back to the ER by ambulance, now severely ill—dehydrated, vomiting profusely, with shaking chills, diarrhea, and bloodshot eyes. On this presentation to the ER, the travel history was elicited and the patient was isolated (though some nurses reported that isolation wasn't immediate and that there was resistance from higher-ups).[8] On September 30, blood tests sent to the Centers for Disease Control confirmed Ebola virus. A week later, on October 8, Thomas Eric Duncan died—the first Ebola case and the first fatality in the United States. Within a week of Duncan's death, two of his nurses became cases two and three of Ebola in the US. (Case four—an American physician who'd worked in Guinea—arrived ten days later at Bellevue Hospital, though the patient went straight to the isolation ward and didn't have the chance to use my office and its lovely sawed-in window with views of the bathroom across the hall.)

Luckily, both nurses in Dallas (as well as the physician who came to Bellevue) were treated early and survived. In the Dallas case, though, scores of people were unnecessarily exposed to Ebola because of the initial misdiagnosis—everyone in the ER, anyone who came in contact with Duncan after he left the hospital, the ambulance workers who brought him back to the ER, any other patients transported in that ambulance, and anyone Duncan's nurses came in contact with. Close to two hundred people had to be monitored for weeks due to the missteps in handling Duncan's case.

As with all medical errors, there was not one single mistake here but many overlapping ones, any of which—if corrected—could have changed the outcome of the case. The initial error—not connecting the travel history with the feverish illness—rightly got the most attention. If those two dots had been connected from the get-go, the patient would have been isolated and treated at a much earlier stage. He might have survived, and his nurses might not have been infected, and two hundred others would not have been pulled into the Ebola net.

The hospital put the blame on the EMR.[9] The nurses' triage template had a field that prompted them to ask about travel history, in order to trigger reminders about necessary vaccinations. Because vaccination is considered a nursing issue, the travel history field was not designed to populate into the screen that the doctor works from. So the physician who was evaluating Duncan didn't know about the travel history the nurse had entered. Score one for error due to the EMR. But of course, he could have—and should have—asked for that bit of information himself, given the well-publicized Ebola epidemic. Score one for diagnostic error on the part of the physician.

Pre-EMR days, before doctors and nurses were chained to their respective and isolated computer terminals, they were squashed into the same physical space and did things like talk to each other. In this antediluvian scenario, the nurse might have turned to the doctor and mentioned the tip-off about the travel history. Score one for error due to poor communication.

As with most medical errors, however, the mistakes and responsibilities in this case radiate in multiple directions. The patient didn't tell the airline—or the hospital—that a week prior he'd helped out a woman in Liberia who turned out to have Ebola. The Dallas 911 system didn't screen calls for Ebola symptoms, as the New York City 911 system did. The ambulance that transported the patient didn't get decontaminated for two full days, allowing more patients to get exposed. The second nurse who came down with Ebola was given permission by the CDC to travel to Ohio to visit her family. These many overlapping errors are frustrating, because each offered a missed opportunity to mitigate or even prevent the error that ended in the death of a patient and the infection of two medical personnel who'd cared for him.

While one can't say that the EMR was the inciting cause of the chain of errors, the fragmenting of information (in this case the travel history) created a fateful fork in the road in this patient's care. The hospital fixed this flaw in their EMR after the event, but the unwieldiness of information in the EMR remains a potent source of future errors.

Exactly one day after I wrote this section on the Dallas Ebola case, I was supervising our walk-in clinic at Bellevue. Late in the afternoon, a kerfuffle broke out at the front desk. A patient was demanding to see a doctor, but the clinic had reached its capacity, and so he was—per policy—referred to the emergency room downstairs. He wasn't happy about that, and it turned out that he was a patient of the medical director, so the top brass got involved. Policies and rank were slung about, triage protocols were debated in the hallway, but at length the administrative issues were ironed out, and the patient finally had his intake with the nurse. A few minutes later the nurse approached me and said, "This patient reports a cough and a fever, and he just came back from Saudi Arabia two days ago."

I'm not a superstitious person, but I couldn't help wondering if having just immersed myself in the case of a patient with fever and recent travel to an endemic country had re-created the real-life scenario not 24 hours later. In this case, the situation of concern was Middle East respiratory syndrome, or MERS.

We'd already avoided the first error of the Dallas Ebola case, as the nurse connected the fever and the travel history and appropriately conveyed that to the doctor (using that old-fashioned technology of talking face-to-face). She'd already given the patient a mask and isolated him in a room by himself, so we'd avoided the second error of the Dallas case.

Now we could take a few minutes to think. My colleague hunted down our infection-control protocol while I scoured the CDC website for the particulars of MERS. In addition to the obvious things like asking a patient about contact with other people who might have MERS, you also have to screen for contact with dromedaries—the single-humped variety— which are the reservoir of the MERS virus. (The two-humped camels appear to be immune.) It's important to ask, for example, if the patient had milked or slaughtered a camel (direct contact) or was merely visiting a camel market or attending camel races (indirect contact). Score one for online databases having better memories for details than humans.

We were just getting our dromedary questions coordinated (as well as our protective gowns and masks) when an investigative team descended on the scene and the bluff was called. The whole thing had been a test. Our hospital was checking to see if our clinic was prepared to deal with "emerging pathogens" that could turn up anywhere, anytime. We fell short on our administrative handling—shunting the patient to the ER could have led to an infected patient unnecessarily exposing others to the virus. Instead, we should have triaged the patient, even if the clinic didn't have the capacity to do a full evaluation. Triage would have determined whether isolation was needed or if the patient could safely go to the ER.

But we were given passing grades on the clinical end—eliciting the travel history, promptly isolating the patient, and then taking the time to access the infection-control protocols and CDC information before beginning the examination of the patient.

It was an effective exercise. All of us had been fully convinced that it was a real case. (The patient had sprinkled in some cinema verité by repeatedly pulling off his mask, arguing with the staff, and pulling rank about knowing the medical director.) We learned about our shortcomings—and about camels—but mainly it emphasized to me just how daunting the task is. A small error, as happened in the Dallas Ebola case, could easily explode into magnified consequences. We were only a hair's breadth from making an analogous error by letting the patient saunter over to the ER, potentially coughing his way past scores of unsuspecting people. It also drove home the point that time to think is one of our most important error-prevention tools, but one that our current state of healthcare seems to conspire to eradicate.

---

One morning, I was sorting through my in-basket in the EMR. This is the collection of any test that I've ever ordered for a patient, any order from a nurse, any note from a social worker, any request for a medication refill, any message from a patient, any note from an intern needing to be signed, any notification that a patient of mine has visited an ER, emails from staff, consultations from specialists—pretty much anything connected to any of my patients or to me.

On one level, the in-basket is an enormous step forward in patient safety. Before the electronic medical record, a doctor had to actively seek out the results of any test he or she ordered. Following up on test results was therefore entirely dependent on the memory or to-do list of each individual doctor. Throw in a late night on call—or a late night partying—plus a few competing phone calls from other departments, three meetings to attend, and a waiting room or ward full of patients, and you can see how things were missed with regularity. And it doesn't take missing much to cause a disaster—a missed mammogram that showed an early cancer, an elevated potassium that could cause a fatal arrhythmia, or a gonorrhea infection that could be passed on to someone else.

The EMR allows test results to be tied to an individual physician. Every single test I order for a patient is automatically routed to my in-basket when it's ready. Nothing can be archived until I've signed off on it. In theory it's a great system but in practice the in-basket is an unwieldy beast. I try to be judicious when I order tests, but even when I'm at my conscientious best there's a constant stream of results to sort through. Clearing the in-basket is a holy grail for my colleagues and me, but it can never happen because there are always more tests rolling in. The in-basket can only go from full to fuller, and sorting through it takes hours.

Taking care of even just a single test result involves more steps than you might think. Usually there is a time lag between when I saw the patient and when the test result shows up in my queue, so in order to evaluate the test result appropriately I have to retrieve the chart for that patient, dig up my last note, and reread what I'd written to remind myself of the patient's clinical situation. If it's something like a blood sugar, I'll need to compare it to previous results. If it's something like cholesterol, I might have to pull up a cardiac risk calculator (which will also require retrieving other necessary information such as age, sex, blood pressure, and tobacco use) to decide what to do with the cholesterol results. Some tests results require me to refer the patient to a specialist. Some results require a medication change, which involves writing and sending a new prescription, plus making a phone call to discuss the change with the patient, who might remember three things she forgot to bring up at our last visit. And then our conversation and treatment decisions need to be documented in the chart. A single test result can take up to fifteen minutes to resolve.

Periodically I'll down three cups of coffee and do a blitz of my in-basket to clear out everything. But the victory is ephemeral, because minutes later another result pops up, and then another. By the next day there are a dozen. Each day that I see patients, more tests are generated. There are days when I envy Sisyphus: at least it's the same stinking boulder he's pushing up the hill every day. For a doctor, it's a sea of boulders, any of one of which—if missed—could come crashing down on one of my patients. Or on me, in the form of a lawsuit.

One day, I was sorting through my in-basket, trying to balance the need for speed with the need to stay focused. I came upon Emile Portero's glucose, which was still astronomically high, despite his elephantine doses of insulin. His decades of diabetes had already cost him one leg and most of his vision. The severe vascular disease associated with his diabetes made his prosthesis fit poorly, so he mainly used a wheelchair now. His kidneys had taken a hit and I worried that dialysis could be lurking on the horizon.

Before I called him about these lab results, though, I wanted to open his chart to remind myself about our last insulin adjustments. Because of his obdurate diabetes and its cascading complications, Mr. Portero was a prodigious user of the medical system. His electronic chart reflected that and took longer to load. Spending even thirty seconds staring at a whirling graphic while there is so much more work to do sends me into a tizzy, so while Mr. Portero's chart was loading, I moved on to the labs of the next patient in my review queue: Hassan Jalloh.

Mr. Jalloh had been diagnosed with diabetes only a year ago, and he was in the throes of completely retooling his life. He'd dumped the white rice, which had been his daily manna. The goat stew was gone. The syrupy baklava was history. Fanta orange soda had been excised. He now whipped up "green juice" in the blender on a daily basis and was a legume poster child. When he was diagnosed the year before, he'd required two medications to control his diabetes. But now we'd been able to discontinue one of them and were in the process of weaning him off the second.

Mr. Jalloh's youthful medical chart loaded much more quickly than Mr. Portero's, so I decided to call him first. "Great news!" I said. "Your sugar is staying down nicely. All your hard work has paid off. I think we'll be able to stop your medications completely." With a disease like diabetes, we don't often have unadulterated good news to relay to our patients, so this type of phone call is as rare as it is thrilling.

Mr. Jalloh was clearly elated too. "That's fantastic," he practically sang into the phone. "This is the first time I've ever gotten good news about my sugar!"

First time?

"You really made my day, Dr. Ofri! I can't wait to dump all my syringes into the trash. Goodbye, insulin!"

Syringes? Insulin? *Uh-oh.*

I realized I had accidentally dialed insulin-dependent, amputated, obese, wheelchair-requiring, nearly blind Mr. Portero, not lentil-toting, kale-convert, rail-thin Mr. Jalloh. (Only in the sterile digitized world of the EMR could two patients so vastly different be confused for each other.) Now I had to backpedal—on two counts! First I had to tell Mr. Portero that I'd made a mistake, mixing him up with someone else. But then I also had to tell him that the good news was a false alarm. His sugar wasn't low at all; it was depressingly—and intractably—high.

I apologized profusely, and we spent the next ten minutes talking about his situation, working to find the baby steps that he'd accomplished and small goals that he could shoot for. I struggled to find something optimistic to tell him, but it was tough.

I'd fallen into the trap of having two charts open at the same time. It's easy to say that I was just being stupid. It's a complete no-no to have two charts open at the same time—I know that! I warn my interns and students about this till I'm blue in the face. And yet here I was doing it, and making an error because of it. I could easily have accidentally prescribed Mr. Jalloh's pills to Mr. Portero and sent them electronically to his pharmacy. Mr. Portero might easily have taken that medication, because he was on so many pills that changed so often that he might not have noticed one extra diabetes medication.

But Mr. Portero's kidneys were in no shape to handle Mr. Jalloh's medication. That one extra medication could have been the straw that broke the camel's back (single-humped dromedary, of course). That one nephrotoxic insult could have been enough to push Mr. Portero's fragile kidneys into dialysis territory.

I recognize that the user (me) was the primary driver of this error, but the EMR also played a role. The EMR is both cumbersome and also ridiculously easy to use. In the paper-chart world it would be impossible to mix up a doorstop chart like Mr. Portero's with a flimsy novella-sized chart like Mr. Jalloh's. In the EMR, it only takes a click.

---

It's tempting to blame nearly everything on the EMR and technology. The frustrations of using these systems loom large in our daily experience (often larger than the many miraculous tasks these technologies can accomplish). Ultimately, though, they are only tools, and we in medicine—with input from patients and society at large—need to decide how these tools are utilized. As Bob Wachter said in his article commenting on the Dallas Ebola case, "We need to take advantage of these marvelous tools, but not forget that they don't practice medicine. We do."[10]

EMRs have done many wonderful things that improve medical care. Just having all the medical records in one place is a monumental improvement over the days of lost charts and misplaced X-rays. And it's certainly a step up from inscrutable handwriting, coffee stains, and remnants of Thai red curry. Additionally, the EMR can allow for quick access to online resources when additional information is needed, instead of running down to the library to look things up.

Another excellent way that the EMR can improve medical care is by enabling analysis of a population. A hospital can, for example, survey all patients with diabetes and figure out who hasn't seen the eye doctor in more than a year, or whose cholesterol is too high. This can help a hospital figure out whether it needs to hire another ophthalmologist or invest in more nutrition education. This type of analysis can also show whether various interventions produce results. If hospitals invest in extra nurses to call patients at home after they are discharged, for example, does this decrease the readmission rate?

But EMRs can also worsen medical care and introduce errors. Cumbersome usability forces doctors and nurses to take shortcuts that can be dangerous. Alert fatigue means that important warnings get lost because they are swimming in a sea of liability-induced minutiae. Diagnosis codes that are driven by billing requirements can distort the diagnostic process. Copy-and-paste ability can lead to voluminous notes that resemble those online "terms of service" agreements that you surely read assiduously.

To me, however, the biggest damage comes from the fact that the computer has centered itself as the most important thing in the exam room, not the patient. It's hard to have a real conversation with one person's eyes bolted to a screen. I don't lament this damage to communication *just* because I think that the schmooze aspect of medicine is the most fun. I lament it because communication with patients is one of the most powerful strategies we have to reduce medical error. It's not the deus ex machina for everything, but nearly every medical error I've reviewed for this book could have been prevented—or would have its harm minimized—had there been better communication between medical professionals and patients. Certainly Jay's case reveals numerous examples of poor communication. The medical staff didn't communicate well in terms of explaining their diagnostic reasoning or the medical treatments. And they certainly didn't do so well on the listening front either when Tara tried to talk to them.

Technology played its role in the errors, too, as staff appeared to give more weight to readings from the machines (e.g., the oxygen saturation monitor that was in the normal range, a chest X-ray that was negative) than to the patient's clinical condition, which was steadily worsening. The so-called objective measurements created an image of the patient that did not at all match the situation of the actual patient lying in the bed. Bob Wachter's comment about technologies and responsibility in the Dallas Ebola case holds true here: "They"—the machines—"don't practice medicine. We do."

It's certainly possible that Jay might have died even if he'd received the most meticulous medical care. He had a severe form of leukemia, after all, and he was infected with a virulent bacteria after undergoing a punishing treatment of chemotherapy—all things that can be deadly on their own, let alone in combination. But there's no doubt that his medical care was undermined by shoddy communication that no amount of technological wizardry could overcome. Communication wasn't the only error in Jay's case, but poor communication compounded the harm every step of the way.

# CHAPTER EIGHT

# THE HUMAN CONSEQUENCES

W hat exactly *do* you do after your husband has died in front of your very eyes?

The frenzy of the code had dissipated by now. Staff streamed out of Jay's room, shedding protective gowns and masks, wheeling out carts and equipment. A housekeeper lugged a mop inside.

Tara had been shunted into the hallway and now stood just outside of Jay's room trying to figure out what she was supposed to do now. She sank back against the wall next to his door. Was she supposed to call someone? Fill out paperwork? Stand there and wait? And who or what was she supposed to be waiting for? There wasn't anything about this in the glossy "Welcome Guide" they'd received when Jay was first admitted. The unbearable hopelessness sapped the last vestiges of muscle function in her legs, and she worried that she might melt down onto the linoleum floor and dissolve into the industrial flecks of brown, beige, and gray.

Tara didn't know what she was supposed to be doing in these post-death minutes, but unfortunately she knew exactly what was happening to Jay in those minutes. She knew precisely what the postmortem care would be, because she'd been there and done that. As soon as the distraught family members were led out of the room, it was the nurses' job to prepare the body. Tara shuddered, knowing what was transpiring on the other side of the wall as she huddled in the sudden solitude. She tried to block out the images from her head, but they came at her relentlessly, obtrusively. Tara could see the nurses wiping off the bodily fluids—the blood, the vomit, the feces. She could see them pulling out the IVs and removing the EKG leads. She hoped they were being gentle, but she also knew that this was merely a job for them. The nurses might easily be talking about their upcoming vacations while peeling off excess tape and gauze from Jay's body. Even if they were performing their tasks respectfully, they might be talking about a date last weekend or commiserating over their onerous schedules, knowing that their patient could not overhear.

Tara could see them rolling Jay first left and then right to ease the vinyl body bag under his stiffening body. While tugging away the blood-stained sheets, they might be laughing at something ridiculous they'd overhead in the cafeteria. A limb might slip over the edge of the bed while one nurse was recommending the new Lebanese place across the street that gave a 15% discount for anyone with a hospital ID. For these nurses, preparing a body was just a job.

But the most harrowing part for Tara was envisioning the final task. There was one last thing for the nurses to do before they could resume their regular work that had been disrupted by the code: they had to zip up the body bag. The zipper would start at Jay's feet. It might catch on the first attempt. The nurses would grimace and give it a more forceful tug. After a hiccup, the zipper would shackle together the first clutch of teeth. Then it would grind unwaveringly upward, gradually entombing Jay's body in white vinyl. The nurses would have to pull up slightly as they rounded the thorax and approached the head. And then, with a final yank, they would zip the bag over Jay's face.

"I knew darkness would finally encase him in that white, airless body bag," Tara said, describing that moment to me. "This was the face I used to caress and kiss and snuggle against. The thought of Jay unable to breathe in that bag started taking my own breath away. I began to suffocate. I thought I was going to die from profound fear and sadness."

Tara couldn't bear to stand on her side of the wall, assaulted by the image of Jay on the other side, suffocating inside the body bag. She would explode if she stayed any longer. There was nothing for her here—nobody and no place. She staggered down the hall and out of the hospital. There was really only one place where she'd feel safe. Only one place where she would be understood—the ER.

Somehow she managed to drive back to her own hospital. She hobbled into the triage bay, collapsing into the first nurse she encountered. "I think I'm going to die," she said. Tara was quickly swooped off to a quiet exam room by her colleagues, who surrounded her with comfort. Someone took her vital signs and then immediately started IV hydration.

"Jay was killed," she told them, sobbing. "No, *murdered!* Jay was murdered." She caught the look exchanged by the doctor and the nurse tending to her, but she persisted. "I'm not crazy," she implored. "They *killed* him." She moaned and wept in the secure presence of her ER family, feeling safe for the first time in what seemed like forever. She was finally with people who wouldn't let her die, even though that was what she ached for.

A nurse injected a syringe into the IV, and from the corner of her eye Tara caught the oily glow of the syringe's contents, recognizing it as Ativan. "Give me only 0.5 mg," she said faintly. "I can't tolerate the whole milligram." Another one of the nurses hugged her, cradling her face as the room narrowed to a black slit, and she fell into leaden, airless sleep.

---

It took Sasha three full days to travel home from China. A missed connection left her stranded in Shanghai, alone at age fifteen, unable to reach her mother, still processing the recent news that her father had been diagnosed with cancer, still coming to terms with the abrupt cessation of her trip. But Sasha had inherited Jay's resourcefulness. She used the emergency credit card her father had given her, figured out how to book a room and get to a hotel, rescheduled her flight, and, seventy-two hours later, arrived stateside—jet-lagged and drained but all in one piece.

Tara was waiting at the airport with as many family members as could fit into the van. She was nearly comatose during the two-hour drive to the airport, needing her family to prop her up, even brush her hair, but she was able to make it known that she wanted to give Sasha time to recount her trip before learning of the terrible news that awaited her. She wanted Sasha to have a respite of normalcy, a moment of being a teenager relishing the accomplishment of a challenging experience that would be a defining milestone in her life— before the anvil of an even more life-defining experience would fall upon her.

On the drive home Sasha unloaded all the stories of her trip, bursting with details both memorable and mundane. She sat in the backseat, tucked between Tara and Tara's sister—a carefully planned arrangement. Sasha chattered about her culinary and linguistic adventures (and misadventures) in China, handing her mother a delicately decorated box of tea as a gift. Sasha described the different members of her host family as well as the suicidal driving techniques favored by city drivers. By contrast, the monastery was peaceful beyond anything she'd ever experienced before. Being with the monks was as intense as it was moving.

Tara's youngest brother was driving the van. The plan was that after an hour, at the halfway point in the trip, he'd give Tara the signal. That's when Tara would shift the conversation. But still, when the raised eyebrows appeared in the rearview mirror, Tara froze. How could she bring herself to collapse her daughter's world? How could she tell her daughter that she wasn't brought home from China because her father was ill. She was brought home because her father was gone. Forever. The goodbye hug that her father had given her at the airport three weeks earlier? That would be it. The last touch of her father. Forever.

Tara agonized in her seat. How could she, as a mother, deliver such pain to her child? At that moment, Sasha reached into her bag and pulled out a parchment scroll from the monastery, with Chinese prayers printed in intricate script. "I got this for Daddy," she said.

Tara couldn't hold off anymore. As she recalled, "I could no longer be a mother; I had to be a nurse." The paralysis of her grief was temporarily shunted aside as the switch to nurse mode clicked inside her. She explained to Sasha about Jay's diagnosis of leukemia and the chemotherapy and the fevers. Tara was careful to keep her verbs in the present tense. She explained why they hadn't told Sasha initially. "We didn't want to tell you he was getting chemo because we wanted you to enjoy your trip," she said. "We figured that you'd come home and Daddy would be bald and skinny and a bit weak."

As she was telling this to her daughter, Tara suddenly became regretful of how aggressively she'd pursued the medical evaluation back when Jay's white count was just slightly low. Her insistence on the bone marrow biopsy was what had given them the early diagnosis of leukemia and a shot at a cure. But it had also delivered Jay into the hell of the medical care that killed him. Had she not pushed the doctors to do the bone marrow, had the diagnosis been delayed by a few weeks, he might be alive now. Although a delay in the diagnosis might have given the leukemia a chance to take hold and all but guarantee Jay's death within months, at least Sasha would have had the chance to say goodbye to her father.

As a trained nurse, however, she had to shunt her own feelings aside. Tara explained to Sasha, using lay terminology, how the fevers and infection overwhelmed her father and that he had more and more trouble breathing. She left out the part about the doctors and nurses doing nothing to help—she didn't want her daughter burdened with that too. "He fought the infection as hard as he could," she said, "but . . . I am so, so, so very sorry to tell you this: Daddy died."

Tara remembers that Sasha's reaction was instant: her face paled and her eyes grew agitated. Her breathing became so rapid that she appeared close to fainting. In the unsparing silence that followed, Tara took Sasha's hand and told a lie. "Daddy didn't suffer at all," she said to her daughter. "It was peaceful and he just went to sleep."

"It was all I could do," Tara told me. "Was I to describe his slow, agonizing demise? Was it fair to make her understand the horrors of asking for help—over and over—and being denied every time?"

Tara told Sasha truthfully how Jay's last words were about how much he loved her and Chris. She told Sasha that she'd read her email to Jay the night before he died and that the colorful descriptions made him smile. She told Sasha that Jay had said how proud he was of her. Sasha clasped the prayer scroll, turning it over and over in her hands during the remaining hour of the drive home, the scroll that she would never be able to give to her father.

Jay's Navy dress uniform, with its four rows of military ribbons, lay smoothed out on the bed. Tara, who had also served in the Navy, knew full well how to assemble a uniform but on the morning of the funeral she could hardly stand, much less coordinate the proper positioning of epaulettes and insignias. Just envisioning the ceremony was overwhelming. The image of the casket cover that would close down on Jay brought back frightening memories of Jay's struggle to breathe. And each time the memory of his agony unfurled in Tara's head, her own breathing would constrict nearly to asphyxiation. She downed an Ativan tab before leaving the house. It was the only way she'd be able to make it through the ceremony.

"As Jay's face became visible to me over the side of the pale-gray casket," Tara recalled of that day, "I was overcome with a profound hollowness. There he was, motionless in his US Navy service dress blues. Still purple and mottled from his fight for life." *Rest in peace* seemed like a cruel taunt. It took every bit of strength to hold herself together as she watched Sasha gently place the scroll of Chinese prayers into her father's arms.

The funeral director moved to close the casket, and Tara suddenly felt the sanctuary begin to spin. She'd hardly eaten in a week and the throbbing emptiness unsteadied her. "I looked at Jay," she remembered, "and began to realize I would never see him in the flesh again." This recognition crashed in on her, and nothing in her surroundings could temper it—not the swell of loving family and friends around her, not the sympathetic religious clergy, not the stalwart presence of Jay's naval colleagues, not even the cocoon of her ER family.

An uncontrolled wail escaped from her and reverberated off the domed ceilings. Tara's legs foundered and she buckled into the side of Jay's coffin. The sturdiness of the coffin, though, kept her from collapsing. "Yet again," she recalled bitterly, "Jay was holding me up when I was weak." A morbid vision flashed through her head, of secreting his stiff, purpled body at home just to keep him close. This seemed no more bizarre than any other aspect of the nightmare that she was living through. "Suddenly, his death was tangible," Tara said. "It was harsh and undeniable. My best friend, my lover, my children's father . . . was dead. He had been killed by people who had no idea that their decisions carried such finality."

Jay's flag-draped casket was carried to the cemetery by a military detail. After laying the casket at the graveside, the servicewomen and -men folded up the flag with crisp, respectful precision while the notes of "Taps" poured mournfully from a Navy bugler. After the smart salutes, a serviceman did a sharp about-face and knelt before Tara. "It was just like you see in the movies," she remembered. He started with, "On behalf of a grateful nation . . ." and that was enough to wrench open the floodgates. Tara did not hear a single word of the recounting of Jay's military honors. She clutched the flag to her chest, tears streaming down her cheeks. Tears not just for Jay's death but for all the years of sacrifice. The never-ending deployments that may have served a grateful nation also served to tear Jay away from his family. The ongoing military commitments denied Jay the precious babyhood years of his children. The endless trainings that helped keep the Navy at the ready also helped keep Jay absent from so many family celebrations and ordinary weekends. Time lost, never to be regained.

What do you say when people ask, "What happened?" Do you sanitize it and offer an easy-to-swallow plotline about the tragedy of cancer? Or do you unload the complicated, uncomfortable, protracted truth, even on well-meaning people who are not expecting a medical tsunami? As a straight-talking nurse, Tara was never much for sugar-coating. So when people asked, she answered. Truthfully.

"The answer wasn't short," she said. Each time Tara told the story, though, she had to relive it. "Each time I told it, I shook uncontrollably," she recalled. "I would be swept away with nausea and penetrating fear." And even when she *wasn't* telling the story, she was still reliving it. "The recurring visions in my head of Jay's dying were actually more unbearable than what I had seen with my own eyes," Tara said.

The anger was overwhelming. All she could think of was having the medical team imprisoned for murder. "I believed they'd committed a crime by knowing he was dying, based on my warnings of his decompensation," she said. "They not only did nothing, but his oxygen was turned *down* just hours before his agonal breathing commandeered his failing body."

Some friends suggested a lawsuit and even gave her names of malpractice lawyers. But such was her state in the days and weeks that followed Jay's death that nothing registered. "I know I jotted down the information," Tara told me, "but when I read the names and numbers later, I couldn't even recognize my own handwriting."

A few weeks after the funeral Tara sat at her mother's formal dining table, swamped with papers. Who knew dying involved so much paperwork? There were hospital bills and insurance forms. Papers from the bank and credit card companies. There were things to handle from Jay's job and his retirement account. There was stuff to sort out with the military and life insurance. Social security and the DMV. Tara had to figure out what to do with online accounts and passwords, with cell phones and email accounts. It was endless.

She couldn't make even the simplest of decisions. "It was like my IQ had dropped fifty points," she said. "I had become almost illiterate as a result of Jay's death." Basic forms were inscrutable. Numbers dissolved and reaggregated on the page like acrid remnants of a hallucinogen. She became afraid to make any decisions, worried that she'd inadvertently trigger some financial calamity by checking the wrong box. She hardly trusted herself to close the refrigerator door, much less calculate insurance payouts.

And of course the school year was just about to begin for Sasha and Chris, so there was the usual avalanche of registration forms and athletic forms and afterschool permissions and PTA requests. Plus the stacks of thank-you notes to well-meaning friends and family for all the offers of support. "Everyone was eager to help," Tara recalled, "but it's too fragile a concept—this dying thing. The house was filled with people and food, yet it never felt emptier."

As she sat at the table that day, drowning in incomprehensible paperwork, her younger brother came into the room. He was a bodybuilder, with biceps and pecs that resembled midsize mountain ranges. But he was tiptoeing now, his enormous hands cupped gingerly around something small and furry. It looked like an injured baby bird. He tried to speak but couldn't. All he could do was to stand before Tara and silently open his hands.

There, in his palms, was a lock of Jay's hair.

It was only six weeks earlier that the extended family had formed an impromptu barber's shop under the maple tree, offering Jay the bittersweet sendoff to the world of patient-hood. Six weeks can be a lifetime for a lawn (and for a patient too). In those six weeks the lawn had been mowed three times, it had served as a parking lot for the swells of visitors and family, it had absorbed the rains of August and the early winds of September. And yet, somehow, this solitary lock of hair had managed to stay nested within the grass.

"As my brother poured Jay's hair into my hands, I thought my heart would fall out of me," Tara remembered. "I felt it sink into my chest, lost forever. I'd thought I was out of tears but I shook and cried, holding this delicate little bird in my hands."

Tara tucked the hair inside the last shirt Jay ever wore and slept with the bundle under her pillow for weeks, inhaling his scent for as long as she could.

---

It took three months for Tara to set foot back in a hospital again. It was the day of her thirty-eighth birthday and she was marooned at home, sinking into the misery of yet another day, when a nurse called, desperate. It was her wedding anniversary that evening and she'd forgotten to block the date. Could Tara please, please cover her shift in the ER?

In some ways it was a blessing—an out-of-the-blue, last-minute coverage request from someone who didn't know that Tara hadn't donned scrubs in twelve weeks. Tara's head nurse wasn't sure if Tara was ready to assume her previous level of nursing—handling codes and trauma—so Tara was "banished" to triage, where she would take vital signs and do the initial intake of arriving patients. Thus she began her painful reentry into the medical world, a forced and discombobulating transformation from being on the patient side of medicine to being back on the provider side.

Tara slowly took on more shifts but found that even the most mundane medical tasks triggered intense flashbacks. Just reaching for a blood pressure cuff rekindled a memory of the monitor at Jay's bedside that registered his escalating heart rate and plummeting oxygen saturation. The croup of his struggle for air echoed in her ears, and she would gasp for breath as her own throat began to constrict. Her neck and jaw were permanently clenched and she ground her teeth incessantly, to the point where two teeth eventually had to be pulled.

Tara found that she was intolerant of physicians who appeared lackadaisical, vocally taking them to task. At the same time she became obsessive over the slightest abnormality in a patient's white count, in case leukemia might be lurking. She got into arguments with other staff over inconsequential matters. On her breaks, she wandered aimlessly through the halls of her hospital. But this triggered memories of Jay's hospital, and then she'd be assaulted by visions of Jay suffocating in his bed, turning from pink to faintly blue to purple to dead. Shaking, she'd reach for the nearest trash can, vomit whatever there was to vomit up, and then stagger back to her post. Each ER shift left her heart racing.

One of her colleagues finally pulled her aside in the ambulance bay, concerned about her state of mind. When she told him about the visions of Jay's death that were plaguing her, he said, "You know, you might have PTSD." Post-traumatic stress disorder.

"This was the first time I'd associated those letters with something other than war veterans or rape victims," Tara recalled. "I felt ashamed to be lumped in with those demographics, and I could barely meet his gaze. But I suddenly understood how Vietnam vets had turned so easily to drugs and alcohol. I would have done anything at this point to relieve my mental anguish." She took down his recommendation for a therapist who specialized in PTSD.

She also decided that she needed to step away from clinical medicine. The day-to-day work with patients was simply too traumatic. Tara heard of an opening as a Clinician Nurse Educator and jumped at the chance. Educating nurses would be something pragmatic that could help improve the situation for patients, and possibly help channel her angst over what had happened to Jay. It seemed like a win-win scenario.

But it turned out to be nothing like that. When cases involving errors and near misses were discussed, the administrators seemed to care only about the hospital's financial liability. "Two things happened to me," Tara said. "First, their apathetic attitude about poor-quality patient care pissed me off and made me sick to my stomach. Second, I lost any doubt about suing the hospital where Jay died."

In the public imagination, a malpractice lawsuit is a dramatic affair in which the injured patient or family gets their day in court, like they do on TV. A compelling snippet of forensic evidence is revealed to the jury and the entire case is resolved with a flourish; justice is done, and the miscreants are punished. In reality, of course, the experience of a malpractice case is far from that. As Tara was to learn, it's an immense and painful slog that rarely offers the salvation that is longed for. She did, however, come to this bruising conclusion: "Nothing at the hospital would change unless Jay's death affected their bottom line."

# CHAPTER NINE

# ON THE CLOCK

Jack Adcock was a boisterous six-year-old from Leicester, a city ninety minutes north of London. On a chilly February morning in 2011, his parents brought him to their GP because he was experiencing nausea, diarrhea, and fever. Because Jack had Down's syndrome, including an associated heart defect that had required surgical repair, he was at particular risk for infection. His GP therefore admitted him to the local hospital, the Leicester Royal Infirmary. On the pediatrics ward, he was under the care of the registrar, Dr. Hadiza Bawa-Garba.

The British medical training system uses a different lexicon than the US system, but a registrar roughly corresponds to a senior resident or a fellow, someone who's had several years of training and would be in charge of a ward. A senior doctor would ultimately still be in charge (an attending physician in US terminology; a consultant in British terminology), but the registrar does the lion's share of the daily medical work.

Dr. Bawa-Garba had six years of pediatrics training, but she had just returned from a thirteen-month maternity leave. Two fellow registrars were out that day, with no one to cover their responsibilities, so Dr. Bawa-Garba had to cover the entire pediatrics ward as well as the ER on her own. Her supervising consultant was not on site; he was seeing patients at another hospital because he hadn't realized that he was on call, so wouldn't be able to get to the Leicester Royal Infirmary until later in the afternoon. The only other doctors on her team were two interns. Additionally, the EMR was down, so all orders had to be done manually, and all test results had to be obtained by individual phone calls.

On admission that morning, Jack was lethargic and febrile. His admission blood tests showed an elevated lactate, which can indicate sepsis or dehydration. Dr. Bawa-Garba examined him in the emergency room and found him to be severely dehydrated. Her initial assessment was that this was from viral gastroenteritis. She treated him with IV fluids, but also ordered a chest X-ray and cultures to rule out a bacterial infection. After receiving fluids, Jack's mental status improved, and later in the day he was noted to be drinking water and playing. This rapid positive response supported the initial diagnosis of dehydration from viral infection.

Because of her two absent colleagues (and lack of coverage for them), Dr. Bawa-Garba was evaluating all the new admissions from the emergency room plus taking care of all the patients on the ward, making her responsible for nearly seventy patients. There was one very serious case of a febrile infant with suspected meningitis for whom Dr. Bawa-Garba had to perform a spinal tap that day.

The EMR being down meant that all the tests took longer to process. Additionally, each one necessitated a phone call to obtain the results, further bogging everything down. Jack's chest X-ray from noon did not get a prompt reading by a radiologist as it typically would have. Dr. Bawa-Garba was able to view the X-ray herself around 3 p.m., and she noted a pneumonia. She ordered IV antibiotics to be added to Jack's treatment. It took about an hour for the antibiotics to be administered.

Jack's blood tests from 11 a.m. weren't available until 4:30 p.m. (one intern apparently spent his entire afternoon shackled to the phone, on permanent assignment to track down test results for the team). These tests showed that the lactate had decreased, though it was still not in the normal range.

At 4:30 p.m., the supervising consultant arrived at the hospital and reviewed all the cases with Dr. Bawa-Garba. This was the first time these two doctors had ever met or worked together. In this system, the consultant does not personally examine every patient, only the more complex ones that require additional oversight. Dr. Bawa-Garba shared with him the results of the blood test showing elevated but improving lactate. Apparently, he did not think she was requesting him to evaluate the patient, so he did not personally examine Jack. And since Jack had been improving with fluids and was now receiving antibiotics for the possible pneumonia, the case appeared to be "tucked in." Attention was paid to the more unstable patients.

At home, Jack normally took enalapril, a blood pressure medicine, because of his heart condition. When Dr. Bawa-Garba wrote the admitting orders for Jack, she correctly excluded that medication because of the boy's low blood pressure. However, she did not explicitly warn the parents not to give the medication. In this hospital, it was permissible for parents to administer a child's medications, so at 7 p.m., his mother gave Jack his usual nightly dose.

Perhaps predictably, this antihypertensive medication caused Jack's blood pressure to plummet, and at 8 p.m. a code was called. Dr. Bawa-Garba and the on-call anesthesiologist rushed to the code and began resuscitation.

Earlier that day, Dr. Bawa-Garba had admitted a terminally ill child, one who had a DNR order in place. Sometime during the afternoon, that child had been examined by a consultant and discharged, though Dr. Bawa-Garba was unaware of this because she'd been seeing the other patients (and the EMR was down). About an hour before the code, Jack had been transferred to that very same room.

So when Dr. Bawa-Garba responded to the code, she initially thought it was the terminally ill child and told the team to stop the resuscitation efforts because of the DNR. It took about two minutes to sort out the confusion, at which point she ordered the resuscitation to begin again. The team worked for an hour, but Jack could not be revived. He was pronounced dead at 9:20 p.m.

---

When I first read about this case, I found the whole story devastating. It was about as horrible a situation as I could imagine. I've been that doctor who has been placed in an impossibly overstretched situation and has made mistakes, and I've also been that parent who's had to entrust the medical care of my children to strangers.

I will never forget the morning I brought my eighteen-month-old son to get a simple surgical procedure—tympanostomy tubes in his ears to prevent his recurrent ear infections. In the predawn hours, the pediatric OR was a cheerful and friendly place. The nurses sang songs and the surgeon pointed out the elephants on his hat while we wiggled a hose of anesthetic in front of my squirming son, trying to sedate him enough to get him onto the operating table.

The minute my son slackened, the OR staff clicked into action. The cheery demeanor dissolved, and the patient was whisked from my arms. In less than three seconds, he was strapped on the table with a mask over his face, preternaturally still, *unhumanly* still.

At that moment, my faith in science plummeted. My decades of medical training, my PhD, my grounding in the scientific method all evaporated in the blink of an eye. The sight of my son—stone-still on the OR table, deathly rigid—completely unhinged my confidence that "everything would be okay." Twenty-three pounds of little boy—race-car pajamas and diaper included—seemed minuscule under the ministrations of five lumbering adults and gargantuan, stainless-steel equipment. And there was nothing I could do to help him.

I remember clenching the arm of the orderly who led me out of the OR. "Make sure my son is okay," I beseeched him. He nodded and reassured me, even though as an orderly he had no role at all in the surgery. But he was wearing blue scrubs, so to me he was part of the frightening medical complex that had swallowed up my son.

And this was all for a minor surgical procedure! So I can only imagine the experience of Jack Adcock's parents, the terrifying bargain of uncertainty that all parents make as they entrust their children to the medical system. You, yourself, are not able help your child so you hand him over to the doctors. There's nothing you can do but trust.

But I can also imagine the experience of Hadiza Bawa-Garba: covering a ward of sick children as well as the admissions piling in from the ER, being woefully understaffed, trying to get test results when the EMR is down, being pulled in a hundred directions at once.

There's no doubt that there were errors in Jack's care, although there was no evidence from the news reports that anyone acted with malicious intent. Jack—whose cardiac condition made him a higher risk patient than an average kid with a fever—probably should have been given antibiotics initially, even if simple dehydration from gastroenteritis was felt to be the most likely cause of his symptoms. There are good medical reasons to avoid giving antibiotics when not necessary, but an elevated lactate raises enough of a concern for sepsis to warrant more aggressive care, knowing that you can always stop the antibiotics in a day or two if all the cultures are negative. Additionally, Dr. Bawa-Garba probably should have flagged Jack as one of the sicker patients for her supervisor to get involved with.

The other errors involved the administration of enalapril by the parents (who hadn't been explicitly told *not* to give it) and the two-minute halt of resuscitation due to confusion over which patient was in which bed. Both of these errors are eminently understandable, but they are errors nevertheless. Additionally, the nurses hadn't checked up on Jack as frequently as they should have, given his condition. The supervising consultant was supposed to have been on-site all day and he should have personally examined a new admission with an elevated lactate, no matter what his resident did or did not emphasize.

If any one of these errors had happened alone, would it have been sufficient to cause a death? It's impossible to say, though we know that most bad outcomes require an aggregation of errors. Prevention of even one or two of the errors might have been enough to save Jack's life. Furthermore, as Lucian Leape pointed out in his earliest writings, even if the proximate cause of an error is a human action, there are nearly always systems problems that made the error possible.

That is surely the case here. If the EMR hadn't been down, for example, all the test results would have been available faster, and Jack would likely have received his antibiotics sooner. Also, a functioning EMR would have freed up an intern to assist Dr. Bawa-Garba with clinical work—such as checking in on the sicker patients—rather than wasting his medical skills at a desk making phone calls. If the scheduling process had been more assiduously monitored, the mistake that caused the consultant to be booked with patients at another hospital could have been uncovered in advance and fixed. If the hospital employed a more rigorous system for monitoring medications that parents administer to their children, a nurse might have been able to prevent Jack's mother from giving him the enalapril.

So although every "error" was made by a human, there are myriad systems breakdowns that made these errors possible. It is abundantly clear that the medical staff were working under conditions that were patently unsafe. The very idea that one doctor could cover the clinical responsibilities of three doctors with any degree of thoroughness is ludicrous. No one can take care of that many patients and do it properly. This seems like a story from the dark ages of medical training, before anyone gave any thought to the relationship between the working conditions of staff and the safety of patients.

In the United States, these issues were decisively galvanized in 1984 by the death of Libby Zion, an 18-year-old college freshman who was admitted to New York Hospital on a Friday evening with fever and agitation. She was given a sedative that likely interacted with the antidepressant she'd been taking, causing hyperthermia and cardiac arrest. There were numerous complicating factors in the case, including the patient's possible cocaine use, which was not revealed to the doctors, and the use of physical restraints to control the agitation. But the issue that Libby's journalist father Sidney Zion forcefully publicized was the unsafe working conditions of trainee doctors.

The intern on this case was working a standard 36-hour shift and was responsible for forty patients. Her only backup was a resident with a scant one year more experience than her. The attending was not required to be physically present in the hospital and his input was limited to a few brief phone conversations. (And as anyone who trained at that time could attest, even that amount of real-time contact would be considered a lot. As a resident, you would *never* call the attending at home at night except in the rarest, direst of circumstances.) The intern, like Dr. Bawa-Garba twenty-seven years later, was responsible for far more patients than could be safely handled, and there was minimal oversight from the senior physician.

The deaths of Libby Zion and Jack Adcock were tragic and heartbreaking. It is not surprising that malpractice lawsuits were considered in both cases.

No one would argue that these patients received ideal medical care. However, malpractice is typically a civil court proceeding, in which one party sues another party and if successful receives financial compensation for damages. But in highly unusual moves, both of these cases went to criminal court.

In New York, a grand jury declined to indict the doctors but issued a scathing report about the poor supervision and unsafe work schedules of the doctors-in-training. It pointed a finger at "the system" as the primary cause of Libby Zion's death, which became the instigator of work-hour reforms in the US.

In the UK, Dr. Bawa-Garba was convicted of manslaughter—a conviction that shocked the medical community. She was sentenced to two years in prison and then banned from practicing medicine for life.[1] She appealed her case and was eventually given a one-year suspension from medical practice instead, but the manslaughter conviction stood. The case roiled the medical community in England, who felt that a single doctor was being criminally scapegoated for the failings of the entire system—severe understaffing, lack of adequate supervision, unreliable EMR. The parents of Jack Adcock were devastated when the lifelong ban was overturned, feeling that their son's death had not been given justice. I'll discuss some of the other ramifications of this case in the next chapter, but here I want to focus on it in terms of how working conditions (hours, supervision, support staff) set the stage for medical error. Even if there were other factors that contributed, there is little doubt that unsafe working conditions played a significant role in Jack's death.

---

In the United States, after Libby Zion's death and the dramatic court case that dominated news headlines, New York State convened the Bell Commission to examine the working conditions of doctors-in-training. Its 1989 report castigated the typical 100-to-120-hour workweek and 36-hour call shifts. It recommended limiting trainees to a maximum of 80 hours per week and no more than 24 hours in a row.

In 2003, the 80-hour workweek standard was adopted by the committee that accredits residency programs, making this mandatory across the US. In 2011, revised regulations limited interns to a maximum of 16 hours at a time (and more advanced residents to 24 hours) and mandated increased attending supervision.

For anyone outside the medical world, these restrictions seem like no-brainers. You wouldn't entrust the brake repairs on your car to a mechanic who hadn't slept; why would you do that with your gallbladder? Sidney Zion famously wrote in an op-ed, "You don't need kindergarten to know that a resident working a 36-hour shift is in no condition to make any kind of judgment call—forget about life-and-death." To him—and to many others—it was obvious that excessive hours led to more errors and that reduced hours would minimize errors. However, many things that seem obvious in medicine turn out to be far more nuanced, rarely resulting in a clarion conclusion that can fit neatly on a bumper sticker.

Our trusty friends at the Institute of Medicine took up the issue of resident work hours in 2009. In a four-hundred-page report, the IOM noted the clear need to reduce workload and the fatigue of doctors and to increase supervision. But it recognized that these efforts to limit work hours could potentially backfire for patient safety. With the new regulations, trainees were getting less time with patients, resulting in a decreased depth of education. Patient care was being turned over to many more hands, increasing the risk of error. Rigidly fixed checkout times for residents, in particular, could have disastrous consequences for patients. Surgical residents reported having to walk out in the middle of their operations. Residents caring for unstable patients were forced to leave the bedside in the midst of their patients crashing.[2]

A 2016 study of surgical residents showed that more flexible work hours could be introduced without increasing adverse events for patients or worsening education for trainees.[3] In 2017, the US accrediting body tinkered with the rules again, increasing the 16-hour cap for interns to 24 hours, though the new guidelines stressed the need for enhanced supervision of these least-experienced doctors. The rules also permitted residents an additional four hours weekly if needed, so that no one would have to walk out on a critically ill patient. Further, the 80-hour workweek would be assessed over a four-week average rather than every week, so that hospitals could accommodate the natural ebb and flow of patient care. Doctors could be available for busier weeks or sicker patients, and those extra hours would be offset during slower weeks.

The alterations of duty hours in 2003 and 2011 allowed for a natural experiment, tracking the behavior and outcomes of residents before, during, and after these transitions. Study results varied, but the overall impression was that residents slept more and felt less fatigued. But they often felt more stressed, more worried about making errors because of the increased number of handoffs that the new schedules compelled. There was no change on scores of depression or well-being. The residents reported feeling less clinically prepared, although there was no change in the pass rate of the medical board exams between 1996 and 2016.[4]

These were observational trials, however, and thus are hobbled by inherent limitations. Lots of things happened between 1996 and 2016 that might have affected medical trainees besides changes in duty hours. In 1996, the Internet was just getting started and the pager on your belt was the high end of technology; by 2016, everyone was carrying the equivalent of a full-fledged computer in their back pockets, with access to every medical database, every textbook, every take-out restaurant, and every mind-glazing digital time-waster.

There were other enormous changes that irrevocably altered the on-the-ground practice of medicine over that twenty-year period—the increased availability of advanced MRI, CT, and PET imaging, the rise of minimally invasive surgery, advances in genetic sequencing and immunotherapy, the development of effective HIV and hepatitis C treatments, the rise of the electronic medical record, and the increasing corporatization of medicine, just to name a few. So it's hard to say for sure that reducing work hours was responsible for any of the effects that were, or were not, seen.

This, of course, is where the Greek chorus begins ululating from the proscenium for a strapping randomized controlled trial—the gold-chaliced standard of research. But randomizing cholesterol pills is one thing; randomizing work schedules within a beehive with as many moving and interdependent parts as a hospital is quite another. Which is why the field has not been overrun with these more robust types of studies. And of course it is impossible to do this "blinded," because every person is well aware of what time they stagger home each night. But a handful of intrepid research groups have attempted this.

A teaching hospital in Boston randomized its ICU interns to a traditional work schedule or a reduced-hour schedule to study whether shorter work hours would in fact lead to fewer errors.[5] All the interns were on call every third night. With the traditional schedule, the intern simply stayed through the night, working into the next day (up to 34 consecutive hours). With the reduced-hour schedule, a night-call intern took over from 10 p.m. to 1 p.m. the next day, allowing the regular intern to go home and sleep. The interns on the traditional schedule ended up working 77–81 hours per week, whereas those on the reduced-hour schedule clocked in 60–63. Later on in the year, the groups were reversed, so that everyone ultimately worked under both schedules.

So what did reducing the hours achieve?

Interns on the reduced-hour schedule made 25% fewer medical errors (as determined by both self-report and chart review) than those on the traditional schedule. In terms of the type of errors, there was little difference between the groups in procedural errors. This reflects the common experience that when you are about to make a cut with a scalpel or puncture a vein with a needle, most of us are able to corral the necessary adrenaline, no matter how tired we are. The biggest difference came in the realm of diagnostic error, where thinking is needed. Interns on the traditional schedule made five times as many diagnostic errors as interns on the reduced-hour schedule. They also made about 20% more medication errors.

Despite this, the outcomes of the patients weren't very different. There was no difference in the mortality rate of the patients, or the length of time the patients spent in the ICU. Nevertheless, these results hint that reducing hours and increasing sleep might mitigate some errors.

Another group of researchers tried an experiment on a larger scale by randomizing 63 internal medicine residency programs across the United States to two different work schedules, one with the standard work-hour limits and one that allowed more flexibility.[6]

Residency programs in both groups had to abide by a maximum of 80 hours per week, but in the standard schedule, interns had to check out after 16 hours and were mandated to have 8 to 10 hours off before they could return to the hospital. In the flexible schedule, there was no daily limit on hours, as long as the total for a week didn't exceed 80. Everyone had to get at least one full day off per week.

Over the course of one academic year, more than 3,500 residents across the United States were tracked. Mortality rates for patients were no different in the two groups, nor was sleepiness in residents, nor the amount of time spent with patients and in educational activities.

Despite some misgivings over these limited data for resident work hours, there is a general consensus that limiting hours to a reasonable level is salutary, even if many disagree on what is considered "reasonable." The one-size-fits-all approach to schedules is probably too rigid, and there seems to be room for adaptation within the 80-hour workweek.

Hospitals, however, still have to function. There are 168 hours in a week, no matter how you slice it. Patients are permitted to be just as sick at night as they are during the day and someone has to be there to care for them. Kidney stones do not check the calendar for federal holidays before they plunge down the ureter. Peanuts do not adhere to bankers' hours when they trigger anaphylaxis. So residency programs have had to come up with all sorts of creative rejiggerings to ensure that nights, weekends, and holidays are all covered. Often these schedules are so complex that it boggles the mind.

After one of the rollouts of work-hour regulations, our hospital instituted a Byzantine schedule to remain in compliance. It designated different residents on different days to be on long call, short call, early call, and late call. There was a night-float system and a weekend-coverage arrangement, and somehow within that Hungarian goulash everyone also had to be scheduled for a full 24-hour period off every week. We attendings were given spreadsheets with a rainbow of color-coded rows to keep track of eight different wards with every permutation of coverage. You needed a PhD in statistics or maybe one in graphic design to figure it out, and I had neither.

I sat in the doctors' station early one Friday morning during the height (or really the depth) of the transition from the old schedules to the new schedules, absolutely dazed, trying to nail down exactly which members of my teams would be present on Friday, Saturday, and Sunday of the upcoming weekend.

The pre-call resident was on her 24-hour *off* day today, because she was scheduled for *long call* on Saturday and would have to come in on Sunday too. Her absence today, though, meant she wouldn't be part of rounds when the new cases from yesterday were presented. That would be a huge gap for her interns (and me), who would be sorting out those patients today without her input.

The interns, on the other hand, would be present today and tomorrow but off on Sunday, because that would be *their* 24-hour period off. Only the resident would be there with me, but she would be tending only to the new admissions from Saturday, not the rest of the patients. Which would mean I would be covering all the rest of the patients—alone—in addition to working with her on the new admissions.

My other team of residents was on *long-call* yesterday. We had to round on their new cases today. But they had to cease taking admissions at 6 p.m. and physically decamp from the hospital by 9:30 p.m. in order for the interns to abide by the 16-hour cap. An *early shift* of night float started taking admissions at 6 p.m., with a *second shift* of night float starting at midnight. All of those night admissions would also be handed off to us today.

I clutched the lists of patients, blinking dumbly, as white-coated interns and residents swirled around me in an antiseptic blur. I felt vertiginous (and frankly senescent) from all the scheduling innovations. Someone, somewhere had to understand the ins and outs of this and was keeping track. Or at least I hoped so. The sheer number of handoffs was giving me biliary colic, and it wasn't even 8 a.m. yet. With all these sick patients crisscrossing between covering interns, early night float, late night float, weekend coverage, short-call teams, long-call teams—the potential for things to go wrong was staggering. Who might forget to check Ms. Cartena's potassium? Who might miss the change in character of Mr. Barsotti's abdominal pain? Who might neglect to convey the rationale for withholding antibiotics from Ms. Gardiner? Which patient's mental status might drift down without anyone noticing?

Yes, I wholeheartedly agreed that residents should get more sleep, but I wasn't sure if this trade-off was benefitting or harming the patients. Each time care was handed off, by definition that care would be fragmented—continuity ruptured, details lost, subtleties muddied. At best, coverage residents were just putting out fires, not proactively caring for the patients—there simply wasn't enough time. An intervention to reduce hours, thus, could paradoxically end up increasing errors by increasing the number of handoffs. And of course I was ultimately responsible—medically and legally—for all of the patients jiggled between my teams and the various layers of coverage. It frankly terrified me.

Up to 50% of adverse medical events can be traced to some kind of error in handoffs, whether it's from one team of doctors to another, or between doctors and nurses, or between any of the members of the medical team.[7] With the current work-hour limits in place, the care of a hospitalized patient could be handed off to the three different physician teams in the first 24 hours (arguably the most crucial time of a patient's stay) and up to ten times over the course of a typical admission. I often think about that classic summer-camp relay race, the one where you had to ferry a tablespoon of water back and forth, handing it off at each end to another member of your team. Whichever team had the most water left at the end won. Each time the care of a patient is handed off to another person, a few drops of water inevitably spill out. The more times you transfer, the greater the opportunity for spillage. It takes exquisite concentration and a true sense of ownership to keep all that restless water in one spoon.

This handoff moment is fraught with potential for error, yet it has never occupied much attention in terms of teaching or error prevention. For most doctors, it has never felt like an integral part of medical care, on par with *real* things like labs, rounds, X-rays, vital signs, and antibiotics. It was just that one-more-little-thing you had to remember to do at the end of your teeming day, along with going to the bathroom, scarfing down some food, and tracking down where you left your keys. Every team, every program, every hospital did the handoff differently. Even within a team, each person had their own style.

I've observed some interns plodding through reams of obsessive detail with their coverage counterpart. I've seen others hand off their list of patients with a quick and casual "NTD" ("nothing to do") while waltzing out the door. Computerized sign-out systems promised more comprehensive handoffs, but the copy-and-paste reflex could not be suppressed, resulting in tomes of repetitive information that resembled Proustian novels both in heft and style. (The reigning philosophy was that you could be castigated for leaving something *out* but not for leaving too much *in*.)

A team of researchers sought to remedy this haphazard mess by creating a standardized handoff procedure that would navigate the perilous balance between concise information and information overload. They then sought to test it on general hospital wards (i.e., not the small, self-contained atmosphere of the ICU).[8]

They created a mnemonic—medical folks are bred, Pavlovian style, to respond to mnemonics—called I-PASS. And while I doubt they'd hired subliminal marketing strategists, I can't imagine they hadn't noted the sub-conscious appeal of I-PASS to cutthroat medical trainees steeped in high-pressure standardized exams.

The key clinical facts the mnemonic instructed the interns to convey for each patient during the handoff were:

*I* for *Illness Severity:* how sick is the patient?

*P* for *Patient Summary:* a succinct nugget of the patient's illness and treatment plan

*A* for *Action Items:* the to-do list

*S* for *Situation Awareness and Contingency Plans:* what to do if *X* happens

*S* for *Receiver Synthesis:* the person taking over gives a quick recap

The study involved 875 residents and more than 10,000 patient admissions. After the new handoff system was implemented, the researchers noted a 23% decrease in medical errors. The decrease in errors was driven mainly by a de-crease in diagnostic errors and errors related to the history and physical. As with the study of work-hour reduction in the ICU, there was no change in the rate of errors related to procedures.

So it seems that handoffs—like most aspects of medical care, it should be noted—can be improved when attention is focused on them. Work sched-ules can similarly be improved with effort and focus. But overall, the jury is still out as to whether the mandatory changes in work hours for trainees have made a difference on a grand scale. Studies that have examined large population databases—Medicare patients, VA patients—over the decades of change in the US have not seen the headline-worthy improvements in pa-tient outcomes that had been hoped for. On the flipside, there haven't been headline-worthy disasters either. But as alluded to earlier, many things have changed in medicine over these same decades, so it may be that there *have been* improvements in patients safety from having fewer yawning doctors, but perhaps these improvements have been offset by adverse events arising from the EMR, or briefer lengths of stay in the hospital, or bacterial resistance to antibiotics.

The one thing these regulations have definitely and profoundly changed is the *culture* of medical training. Residents were called "residents" precisely because they used to reside full time in the hospital. With each set of work-hour regulations this has devolved into what many derisively refer to as shift mentality. Older physicians pooh-pooh the younger doctors who don't take sufficient ownership of their patients, prioritizing the call of the clock over the call of clinical care.

It is always tempting to condemn newfangled regulations and pine for the "days of the giants." Of course, there's always a bit of accidental idealization in our memories. Every era had its sprinkling of giants, no doubt, but mainly there were legions of ordinary trainees struggling to keep abreast of the clinical and logistical challenges that were thrown to them. Different eras cannot be compared, at least not in any blithely simplistic manner.

Criticism trickles down the hallowed hallways of academic medicine, and the grousing rises to a fever pitch as each new set of regulations is rolled out. Some of the critiques are valid and I hope that vociferous discussion continues to greet every new rule. But there is also a good deal of outright whining. Changing the "gold standards" insidiously suggests that the previous gold standards—those by which *we* trained—were somehow flawed. This represents a not-so-subtle threat to our sense of self, and we rally our defenses.

I admit I am not immune. It seemed that no sooner had I broken through the finish line of residency than the rules were changed. Days off to compensate for weekend call? Leaving before every last patient was "tucked in"? Missing attending rounds when your cases were being presented? Blasphemy! How dare they change those bedrock rules ex post facto?

I'm sure my own attendings were equally appalled at the wimpy rules of my training but it seems that we just can't help ourselves. It's a reflex. Our instinctive resistance to change reflects not just nostalgia, but the fact that medical training sets social, clinical, and moral barometers by which decades of professional and personal life are gauged. These brief years imprint a personal definition in a manner not seen in many other fields; you rarely hear MBAs or accountants clucking about crumbling standards and the days of the giants. For them, training was just training. For doctors, though, training is the forging of a lifelong identity. It is who we are.

In medicine, we always have to be aware of unintended consequences. With all the attention paid to resident work hours, no one really thought much about how things would change for the attendings who were supervising those trainees. Each time a limitation on residents' hours was rolled out, someone had to fill in the gaps. Residency programs didn't double in size with the new rules, so the existing residents were quickly stretched thin by intricate scheduling, and that someone to fill the gap often turned out to be the ward attending.

Gone were the days when attendings graced the ward for two hours per day to wax academic over the handful of new admissions. Now they had to be present all day, every day, including weekends, writing daily notes on all the patients. For many attendings, life started to feel like internship all over again—chaotic days, long hours, sacrificed evenings and weekends. There were many months during this time when I was responsible for up to forty patients at a time. It felt patently unsafe. I often thought about the intern who had cared for Libby Zion and carried a similar-size load. I had more than a decade of clinical training beyond what she had, and still it was nearly impossible to manage. Every single day was suffused with a panic that something, somewhere, sometime could go horribly wrong. I think now about Hadiza Bawa-Garba covering a full ward and an ER essentially on her own. To me, it's shocking that Jack Adcock and Libby Zion were the *only* casualties of those circumstances.

Our hospital eventually realized that our situation was untenable. It increased the attending staffing on the wards so that each would cover only one team of residents instead of two. This decreased the patient load to a more manageable size, but it took time and did not come cheap.

No matter how we slice it, the days of residents living in the hospital are gone. That round-the-clock arrangement worked only because of the more leisurely pace of medicine a few generations ago (as well as the fact that most residents were married men with wives at home to handle life's logistics). Back then, patients commonly stayed in the hospital for weeks at a time, much of which was gentle convalescence. Now, advances in outpatient treatment have meant that the patients who actually get admitted to the hospital are far sicker than in years past, and the financial pressures mean that they remain for ever-shorter periods of time. The breakneck pace of admissions and discharges of these more acutely ill patients has made extended shifts of 36 or even 24 hours indefensible. The safety of both patients *and* doctors is at risk.

Some doctors will continue to pine for the days of the giants, but there is no turning back the clock. And even the giants had to sleep. No matter what system we use, we have to face the fact that at some point in the day or the week or the call cycle, doctors *must* go home, and care *must* be handed over to someone else. Administrators will have to keep experimenting with different scheduling contortions to deal with the inflexible nature of the 24-hour clock; all will have drawbacks, and some will have advantages. We should be constructive—and vocal—in our critiques of each round of changes, but we have to resist the reflex to say that the way *we* trained is the gold standard by which current systems should be judged. Better to direct our energy toward making the octopus of a system work. It's what every generation of doctors and nurses has had to do. Rose-colored glasses only make the challenges harder to see.

One area that has largely gone under the radar is the working condition of nurses. Because of chronic staffing shortages, many nurses end up working overtime. In some hospitals, what is meant to be a stopgap measure has become standard operating procedure.

In a survey of 11,516 nurses, those who worked more than the standard 40 hours per week reported 28% more medication errors.[9] They also experienced 28% more needlestick injuries to themselves.[10] Hospitals often find themselves in a bind because of mandated nurse-to-patient ratios. If they fall short, they either have to push their own nurses to work overtime or hire per diem nurses from outside agencies, who may not be familiar with the hospital routines. Both situations are setups for medical error.

A study of more than 232,342 surgery patients examined nurse-to-patient ratios and mortality. To no one's surprise, the heavier the patient load per nurse, the higher the mortality rate. The researchers calculated that for every additional patient added to a nurses' roster, the odds of a patient dying within 30 days increases by 7%. Nurse burnout goes up by 23%.[11]

A subsequent study drilled down into the details of a single hospital, examining day-to-day and shift-to-shift variations in nursing staffing.[12] The researchers specifically chose a hospital that was recognized for having high-quality care and adequate staffing of nurses. They examined 197,961 patients and found that, at baseline, the mortality at that hospital was lower than would be expected for the illness severity of the patients. But even within this excellent hospital, mortality increased on wards that fell short on nursing staff. The researchers were able to calculate that mortality increased by 2% for *each individual shift* that fell below target levels for nursing staff.

Moreover, they noted that mortality also increased by 4% per shift when there was high patient turnover—admissions, discharges, transfers. These events require significant nursing time, often at the expense of the other patients on the ward. This study underscores that adequate nurse staffing is critical and that staffing needs to be adjusted upward at busier times and for sicker patients. Skimping on nursing is a patient-safety hazard.

There are two other work-hour quirks that have the potential to increase medical error—the July effect and the weekend effect. The July effect, in particular, has assumed ignominious legendary status. And why wouldn't it? July 1 is the start of the medical calendar year. Imagine a flotilla of off-the-boat medical students, ink still dripping from their diplomas, now deposited at your bedside with needles, scalpels, and prescription pads in hand. And of course it's not just those tenderfoot interns with their prepupal clinical skills to worry about. The resident in charge of your team was an intern a mere 24 hours earlier. The nephrology fellow setting up your dialysis just finished being a resident. Luckily, though, they are all being supervised by attendings. (Of course, a slice of those attendings had doffed their resident white coats only hours earlier . . . ) Hence the word on the street: don't get sick in July.

The data on this have been mixed. While we don't see phalanxes of patients mowed down on their gurneys when the calendar turns the page to July 1, there is still certifiable cause for concern. The influx of doctors lacking on-the-ground clinical experience coupled with the exodus of doctors versed in how the system works makes for a perfect storm. The largest review of the data examined 39 studies that tackled this problem.[13] Many of the studies weren't as rigorous as they could have been, limiting our ability to tease out specifics. Nevertheless, a number of studies suggested that errors, inefficiencies, and mortality rates do nudge up at the beginning of the academic year. Many studies did *not* show these effects, but still, attention does need to be paid to this uniquely vulnerable time. Other high-risk industries, such as nuclear power and aviation, do not have this bizarre phenomenon of a significant chunk of experienced professionals exiting stage right, with an equal number of greenhorns entering stage left, all on the exact same day.

Luckily, newbie interns are piercingly aware of their shortcomings (even more than you are, trust me) and border on obsessive-compulsive in their hypervigilance. A rookie intern on the wards is probably the most anal-retentive specimen known to medical science. Every detail on their scut list is triple- and quadruple-checked with maniacal—though admittedly imperfect—rigor.

Most hospitals are cognizant of this tidal wave of inexperience and take precautionary measures, such as doubling up on supervisory oversight, decreasing patient loads, and offering simulation training so that new interns can cut their teeth with actors and/or plastic models (for procedures) rather than on the real thing. More on that later.

One thing that is not routinely done, unfortunately—and that could likely offer significant protection for patients in July—is to increase nurse staffing during that transition period. Hospitals struggle to achieve adequate nurse staffing during the best of times, and they don't have the resources to double up in July. From a patient-safety perspective, though, this is penny-wise-but-pound-foolish.

On the plus side of the July upheaval, there is also some thought that the wave of newness can have benefits for patients, bringing fresh eyes and a burst of investigative zeal. Reevaluating complex cases from scratch is one of the best ways to catch diagnostic errors. As I learned so painfully when my colleague found the anemia that I hadn't noticed in Ms. Romero—the anemia that turned out to be cancer—fresh eyes are of incalculable benefit. Additionally, interns tend to pepper their residents and attendings with endless questions. These often seem simplistic, reflecting their embryonic knowledge base, but in fact they force their superiors to dissemble the logic of their decision-making. This is another crucial way that errors are uncovered.

Ranking up there in hospital lore with the July effect is the weekend effect. Mortality rates tend to be higher for patients admitted on weekends or holidays.[14] Hospitals typically run with a more skeletal staff on weekends. Specialized services are either unavailable or require waiting until the interventional radiology technician or the perinatologist is roused from sleep and makes the drive from home. So it's not surprising that time-sensitive emergency cases experience more errors and adverse outcomes on weekends.

Of course, it may not necessarily be the staffing that's the cause of the worse outcomes. It could be the acuity. After all, who makes the trek to hospitals and emergency rooms on weekends? The sickest, most urgently ill patients. The more mildly aggrieved usually wait until Monday. So it's possible that the higher number of adverse events seen on weekends relates to sicker patients with more moving parts and thus more opportunities for error.

These factors can be difficult to tease apart but it seems that illness severity is likely the primary driver of the weekend effect. (Patients admitted to the hospital at night may also have higher mortality because of increased illness severity.) With this knowledge, hospitals might consider *increasing* resources on weekends, holidays, and nights rather than decreasing them, as is currently the case. Cost, though, is usually the final arbiter of scheduling.

There's no doubt that doctors' and nurses' work schedules affect the rate of medical errors and adverse outcomes, although the data are less crystalline than most of us would like. While we can't say whether Libby Zion or Jack Adcock would be alive today if their medical teams had been working under more reasonable conditions, but it is probably true that there are fewer errors, on average, when doctors and nurses aren't stretched beyond capacity.

Many of the seemingly obvious solutions, unfortunately, have the potential to usher additional errors into the mix because of unintended consequences. But it would be foolhardy to throw up our hands and give up. We should continue to tweak the system to see how it can be improved. We should point out when profits are prioritized over safety, such as with insufficient nurse staffing. Most important, we have to be honest about the twin realities of scheduling: every doctor and nurse has to sleep at some point, and new trainees have to be continually absorbed into the system. Until we have AI-perfected robots that never sleep, get sick, retire, die, or give up and go to law school, we have to work within a system that will always have gaps that need to be covered.

The solutions require a commitment on the part of the healthcare system to ensure that staff are not treated like indentured servants. But it also requires that medical staff reshape how we think of ourselves. The giants who loom so large in our collective consciousness were rugged individualists, battling the rigors of patient care with sheer strength of will. But medicine has changed, and what passed for strength in that era now smacks of foolhardiness. Medicine is a team sport now; complex illness requiring intricate and multifaceted treatment cannot be safely treated by the lone heroic doctor or nurse. Importantly, though, we have to imbue in our trainees the key value that working as a team still requires ownership. If group effort permits responsibility to diffuse, then we end up with a case like Jay's, in which no doctor or nurse stepped up to the plate and assumed ownership of a crashing patient. Such a balance between individual responsibility and team medicine can be achieved, but it can only be done with explicit attention and conscious modeling from the top down.

CHAPTER TEN

# WHAT YOU SEE

The young man stormed into the midst of a medical team congregated at a doctors' station in a back corner of the emergency room. "What are you guys doing?" he demanded, holding up his pink-clad toddler. "My baby's choking, and you guys aren't doing anything!" The ends of his cornrows slashed against his gray hoodie sweatshirt as he spoke angrily to the medical team. This particular doctors' station was out of public view, set behind a staff workroom, so it was clear that the man had crossed through areas that were typically off-limits to patients. As soon as he yelled his opening statement, every person on the team, who were nearly all female, froze.

Ekene, the medical student, looked on with alarm. An "angry black man" invading the doctors' space—this wasn't going to end well. As a medical student, she didn't feel qualified to assess the medical merits of the situation, but as the only African American person among the white doctors, she was acutely aware of the fraught dynamics.

To the best of Ekene's limited clinical acumen, this did not appear to be an acute emergency—the child seemed to be coughing rather than choking. Ekene toyed with the idea of stepping forward and offering to accompany the father and daughter back to their room and begin the medical evaluation. This could potentially calm the situation. But she was lowest on the totem pole and she knew it wasn't her place to take charge.

The highest person in the medical hierarchy at the moment was the ER fellow, and she assumed control. "Go back to your room, sir," she said calmly but with clear authority. "We'll be with you in a moment."

The father edged a few steps away but remained disconcertingly close. Close enough that no one moved a muscle. As the minutes ticked by, the tension ratcheted up. Ekene's eyes tracked back and forth between the father

129

and the medical team, all seemingly cemented in place. Who was going to blink first?

"Fuck you all," the father finally spat, turning on his heel. "I'm just going to take my baby out of here and go somewhere else."

The ER fellow didn't hesitate. "Call Security," she snapped. "Don't let that man leave."

---

When I first heard this story from Ekene, I thought about it in terms of the bias that runs through medicine—both for patients and for staff. In writing this book, however, I've also started to consider the incident in terms of medical error. Ekene was not part of the eventual medical evaluation of the toddler, so she never learned the final diagnosis and treatment, but I've often wondered how it played out with the ER fellow and the patient. The doctor is a human being too and could easily have been rattled by the encounter, or resentful, or distracted. She may have exhibited unconscious racial bias toward the father that leeched over toward the daughter. Or maybe not. She might have performed a more cursory physical exam, or entertained a narrower differential diagnosis, or prescribed a lower-level treatment. Or maybe not. I do not know what happened, and the medical care may have been perfectly excellent. But the situation was, at the very least, a less-than-ideal backdrop within which to begin diagnosis and treatment. It's not a stretch to contemplate that medical error might be higher in these types of charged situations.

Additionally, in this particular encounter there might be biases beyond race that could affect judgment. Many of the biases intersect, even conflict. Was this ER confrontation primarily about a black person challenging a group of white people? Was it about a man acting aggressively toward a group of women? Was this about a patient breaking the unwritten rules of doctor territory? Was this a clash of a white-glove institution sitting in the midst of an economically disadvantaged community? There are so many elements beyond the child's actual symptoms that could have impacted this particular interaction.

There's no avoiding the fact that bias, particularly racial bias, is a potent force in medicine. Maternal mortality, for example, is almost three times higher for African American women than for white women in the United States.[1] There are disparities in outcomes for diabetes, cancer, and heart disease. Socioeconomic factors play a role, no doubt, but significant disparities remain, even when economic differences are factored out.[2]

Explicit discrimination may be less overt than in generations past, but implicit or unconscious bias is still entrenched.[3] Even doctors and nurses who are the most egalitarian specimens of their generation can still demonstrate unconscious bias.

The effect on patients can be difficult to measure in the clinical setting because it's not the type of situation amenable to the usual randomized, double-blind, placebo-controlled trial. But there have been a number of thought-provoking studies in lab settings that suggest that bias could increase medical error. In one such study, doctors were given case studies and asked to recommend treatment. The clinical scenario was identical in all cases (symptoms of a possible heart attack), only the race of the patient was varied.[4] In what is a regretfully unsurprising result, doctors recommended more appropriate (and more aggressive) treatment for white patients than for black patients, even though the clinical situations were identical. This doesn't prove that bias causes medical error, but both diagnosis and treatment were impaired for the hypothetical black patients in this study.

As part of the study, these doctors also took tests to measure both implicit and explicit bias. Interestingly, it turned out that it was the degree of *implicit* bias that correlated most strongly with poorer treatment of the black patients. This was evident even with doctors who showed no bias on tests of *explicit* racial bias. At the very least, this study suggests that even doctors who do not consciously feel affected by the race of their patients can still harbor implicit racial bias, and that this implicit bias may be a driver of unequal medical care as well as medical error.

There are some data to suggest that more diversity in the medical workforce could improve outcomes. In one intriguing study from California, 1,300 black men were randomly assigned to either a white doctor or a black doctor. The doctors—who did not know that the study was about race—were told to encourage their patients to get a flu shot and undertake screening tests for diabetes, cholesterol, hypertension, and obesity. Those patients who were assigned to black doctors were far more likely to agree to the health screening tests.[5]

The possible factors at play—trust, communication, cultural awareness, practice style, preconceptions—are too complex to dissect here, but studies like these offer hints that increasing workforce diversity might improve patient safety, particularly in the realm of diagnostic error.

When Ekene told me the story of the man and his toddler in the ER, I asked her whether she thought the doctors on her team were being racist. This was a complicated knot for her to untie, because these doctors were her *team*. She worked with them intensively, liked them personally, and deeply appreciated how generous they had been with their medical knowledge and encouragement. These were role models—strong women—whom she looked up to. And yet . . .

And yet, she witnessed their automatic reaction to a black man being on their turf. "'Racist' is not a term I use lightly," she said, clearly choosing her words diplomatically. "But I guess I hadn't been aware of the strength of their bias." When the father stormed into the doctors' station, Ekene saw fear and concern in his actions; her fellow physicians saw aggression.

Ekene described her complicated sense of kinship with the father. On the one hand, their lives had nothing in common. She had several Ivy League diplomas under her belt and was attending one of the top medical schools in the United States. This young father was living in a poor, urban neighborhood, relying on charity medical care.

On the other hand, Ekene observed, "that father and I look the same to the outside world." She talked about how she, like other black doctors, was often assumed to be a technician or clerical worker. There is certainly suggestion of racial bias in how society responds to doctors who've made medical errors. Consider the case of Dr. Hadiza Bawa-Garba from the previous chapter. She was convicted of manslaughter in England for the death of Jack Adcock, the six-year-old boy with Down's syndrome who died from septic shock. She was initially banished from medical practice for life. Although the lifetime ban was overturned on appeal, the manslaughter conviction remained.

Two years after Jack's death, a British transplant surgeon, Dr. Simon Bramhall, was found to have branded his initials on patients' livers with an argon laser during surgery. It's not known how many times he did this, but two cases came to light when the patients underwent a second surgery and the initials were discovered. Although the branding caused no medical harm to the livers, the patients were horrified when they learned of it. For this transgression, Dr. Bramhall was fined the equivalent of $13,000 and sentenced to a year of community service.[6]

The discrepancies in these cases shocked many medical observers. In Dr. Bawa-Garba's case, Jack's situation was clinically complex with legitimate diagnostic uncertainty and several plausible approaches that could be reasonably debated. Additionally, there were a number of external factors that might have tripped up even the most conscientious medical professional—having to cover the patient load of two other doctors, the EMR being down, the patients having switched rooms. While there were definitely errors in Jack's care, by all accounts there was no indication of proactive malicious intent.

By contrast, in Dr. Bramhall's case, there wasn't a hint of gray. There isn't any logistical challenge, no diagnostic uncertainty, no overburdened schedule, no clinical conundrum that could inadvertently lead to a doctor's initials being branded on a patient's internal organ. This was a conscious, premeditated, and unethical action, even if it didn't cause any medical harm. Yet Dr. Bramhall got off with a fine and a bit of community service, while Dr. Bawa-Garba was convicted of manslaughter and initially banned from practicing medicine for life.

Dr. Bawa-Garba is a black Muslim woman, originally from Nigeria, who wears a headscarf. Dr. Bramhall is a middle-aged white man who grew up in England. While it is not possible to prove, there is certainly a sense that racial, ethnic, and gender bias might be factors in the vast discrepancy in these cases.

Of course none of this changes the fact that a six-year-old boy died and that his death was possibly preventable. Regardless of the circumstances, the final outcome was that a patient suffered grievous, irreversible harm at the hands of the medical system. Jack's parents were secondary victims who suffered agonizing harm from what transpired in the hospital. It may feel indecorous in the face of such a tragic death to parse the indignities experienced by the doctor, but it is crucial to recognize that *how* we deal with medical error has potent ramifications for whether and how future errors can be prevented. If blame is incorrectly apportioned, or if there is bias in how penalties are meted out, medical workers are much more likely to hide errors and near misses. Such secrecy only serves to make medical care even more dangerous for patients.

---

"In a cardiac arrest, the first procedure is to take your own pulse," wrote Samuel Shem in his satirical novel *The House of God*. It's advice that is relevant in all tense situations, especially ones in which stereotype, bias, and gut reactions can have lasting implications for both medical error and its aftermath. And it's equally important to check the pulse of the others around you. What is everyone else responding to?

Reflecting back on the encounter in the emergency room some years later, the medical student Ekene told me that she wished she had taken the initiative to help the father and possibly defuse the situation. "I no longer take for granted," she said, "that we doctors have it right." This is an Rx that many of us in the medical profession could stand to benefit from. She began exploring the experiences—both bitter and excellent—of friends and family at the hands of the medical profession. "I seek out those stories now," she said.

It crossed Ekene's mind that if she'd walked into the emergency room as a patient, maybe in a crabby mood because of her illness or the six-hour wait, these doctors whom she genuinely respected might treat her the same way they'd treated that father. She might have received flawed or substandard medical care.

But being on the doctors' side of things was equally complicated. During the confrontation in the ER, Ekene experienced an awkward dissonance. Was she first and foremost a medical student, part of the clinical team that was being accosted by an angry patient? Or was she experiencing this primarily as an African American, witnessing the white community prejudging a black man's intentions? And what about the issue of being a female facing a man who feels entitled to challenge the authority of women in charge?

Layered on top of these complications were the power dynamics that also played out in contradictory ways. She was part of the powerful group—the doctors—but as a medical student she was singularly powerless. To the father, she looked like one of "them." To the other doctors on the team, however, a medical student might just as well be part of the furniture. When I reflect back on the tense encounters I've observed over the years—a surgeon screaming at a nurse, a hospital employee confronting an angry patient, a resident dressing down a student—it's always the *other* person who's saddled with the blame.

Even if the person who made the outburst ultimately recognizes the inappropriateness of his or her own behavior, it's somehow the other person who "provoked" the outburst: the nurse gave the wrong instrument, the patient was acting aggressively, the student's work was shoddy. There's always a ready explanation.

Our very human egos demand a mitigating context for our ill-advised actions. These justifications always seem objective because we *know* that we are not racist, or sexist, or homophobic. We are good people and we have chosen to work in a profession dedicated to helping others, right? How could our actions possibly reflect bias?

"When one's own behavior can be construed as negative," researchers Debra Roter and Judith Hall astutely noted in one of their analyses, "the person is particularly inclined to blame it on the other person."[7] Holding back on that blame is a tall order for individuals singularly steeped in the hierarchy of healthcare, but it's a first step in pulling back the bias that so infects our field and jeopardizes the health of our patients.

Addressing bias is a priority in the medical field now, at least a professed one. Resources, though, have not caught up to the rhetoric yet, and frankly I doubt they ever will. Turning a battleship is both an arduous and an incremental process, and certainly offers no help in the moment, which is when these crises typically occur. For better or worse, this leaves much of the issue of addressing bias in the hands of the individuals in the trenches.

Individuals can't fix all of society's ills, but in the moment we individuals can certainly "seek out those stories." What might have happened, for example, if that ER fellow, when confronted by the angry father, had simply asked, "What's going on with your baby?" This would not necessarily have undone the hours of frustration and certainly not repaired centuries of institutionalized racism. But at the very least it would have dialed down the temperature and decreased the risk for medical error. An explosive situation might have turned into a neutral, ordinary one. And if the doctor had been willing to listen honestly to the answers, there might even have been a chance that this could have been a positive experience for all parties involved.

For all its technological innovations, medicine remains an intensely human field: illness is experienced in human terms and medical care is given in human terms. We humans bring along our biases and stereotypes—that is true—but we also bring along our ability to communicate and to listen. We will, of course, never achieve perfection in our interactions with others or in our medical care. No matter how determined we are to be fair and conscientious with everyone, there will always be times when we fall short. But if we take the time to listen—genuinely—we'll at least have the opportunity to peek into the lives of our fellow imperfect humans and attempt to deliver the best medical care possible. We may not be able to step into others' shoes, but we can slide onto the bench next to them and follow their gaze. We can stretch a bit more than usual and attempt to see what they are seeing. This may not be high-tech, but it might very well be our most powerful tool for chipping away at the entrenched bias that jeopardizes medical care.

Thinking back to Jay's case, I wonder how things might have transpired if anyone on his medical team had taken the time to slide onto the bench next to Tara, to follow her gaze and attempt to see what she was seeing. Even if the medical outcome didn't change (though it might have), that small act might have averted a lawsuit. But as things played out, no one really saw Tara's point of view, and her voice—that of a woman, and "just a nurse," at that—was essentially ignored. Losing your voice is a familiar experience for many people in groups that have been historically discriminated against.

Filing a lawsuit can be a way to regain that voice.

# CHAPTER ELEVEN

# I'LL SEE YOU IN COURT

The idea of a legal redress for medical errors dates back almost four thousand years to the Babylonian Code of Hammurabi. It was a strict code, at least if the patient was a person of means: "If a surgeon performs a major operation on a nobleman with a bronze lancet and caused the death of this man, they shall cut off his hands."[1] Surgeons today are surely relieved that modern malpractice penalties center on financial compensation rather than amputations, but King Hammurabi laid down the idea that the doctor bears responsibility if medical care harms the patient. Additionally, Hammurabi developed the beginnings of a trial, with a panel of judges hearing the case, witnesses providing sworn testimony, judgments handed down in written form, and the option to appeal (to the king himself, of course).

The first malpractice case in the United States was in 1794 and focused on breach of contract rather than medical wrongdoing. A doctor promised to perform a surgery "skillfully" and evidently did not, causing the death of a patient. The patient's husband sought redress for breach of contract and won. It took another half century before the idea of "standards of care" came into being, setting benchmarks for what medical care should be. The formation of the American Medical Association in 1847 was largely focused on the idea that there should *actually be* standards of medical care.

In order to prove malpractice in the modern legal system, four criteria must be met:

1. There is an actual doctor-patient relationship (that is, you can't sue any random doctor; it has to be one who has actually taken care of you).
2. The doctor did not adhere to the standards of medical care.
3. The doctor's substandard care was, in fact, the cause of the patient's injury.
4. The patient's injury resulted in quantifiable damages.

The second and third points are the meat of most malpractice cases. Lawyers have to prove not only that the doctor did not render the best medical care, but that the negligence actually *caused* the injury. In practice it can take years of investigation to work this out before a trial can even begin. Lawyers from both sides have to formally question the doctor, the patient, expert witnesses—what is known as the deposition process—in order to figure out if standard-of-care was indeed violated and if the doctor's actions indeed caused the harm.

This process is extraordinarily expensive—requiring money for lawyers, expert witnesses, researchers, independent reviewers, court reporters, and videographers to film the depositions. This can add up to hundreds of thousands of dollars before anyone even sets foot in a courtroom. For this reason, malpractice lawyers are exceedingly selective about which cases they take. Most of the lawyers I spoke to said they have to turn down the overwhelming majority of the cases that patients bring to them. These lawyers work on contingency; that is, they get paid only if they win. Thus, they won't even touch a case unless they are confident it is winnable (all four criteria are met) and that the payout for damages will cover their costs and also provide worthwhile sums to the patient and, of course, to the lawyer. This is where the fourth point—quantifiable damages—becomes critical, since it is these damages that decide what the financial penalty will be. If the patient suffered only a broken toenail (even if the doctor's negligence clearly caused this damage), the payout will not cover the colossal costs of pursuing the case. Lawyers, therefore, usually take only cases in which a patient has been severely harmed.

Jay's case seemed to qualify: Tara felt she could prove that the medical team was negligent in its care of Jay and that this negligence caused the harm. The harm was indeed severe. A lawyer agreed and took on the case.

As the key witness, Tara would have to testify in court. She wanted to be sure that she knew her stuff, so she prepped in the same way she'd prepared for her nursing exams—exhaustively immersing herself in the material until she could recite it backward and forward. By her own account, she became obsessed with the details, of knowing every precise fluctuation in oxygen saturation. But reliving the details, over and over again, was traumatic. "Having to memorize every moment of Jay's death so that I could testify accurately," Tara said, "tore a fiery hole through my heart."

It took a toll on her physical health too. Normally a slim 115 pounds, Tara weighed one hundred pounds at the time of Jay's funeral. She had to borrow clothes from her daughter since none of hers fit. Two months later, she looked down at her belly one day and could see the pulsing of her aorta, the vessel that rests against the spinal column. Her weight was 92 pounds by then. Even sweatpants slipped off her hips.

Tara soon learned—like most people who pursue a malpractice case—that a lawsuit does nothing to heal the pain. On the intellectual side, suing might offer a sliver of gratification in terms of exposing the facts, but on the emotional side, it's more akin to bandaging a wound with sandpaper. One day, while driving on a bridge above a river, Tara was gripped with a vision of driving over the edge. She could see her car sailing through the air, crashing through the surface of the water and sinking. "I imagined myself sitting calmly, waiting for the water to engulf me so that I would cease to exist. Perhaps my kids would be better off. Hopefully, the police would assume I was texting and driving or, maybe, after checking my medical records, that I'd had a longer run of tachycardia causing me to lose consciousness. This way, there would be no mention of suicide, and my kids wouldn't have a problem getting my life insurance."

Tara persevered, though. She had to. She felt this was the only way to get any sort of justice for Jay. She also felt she had an ethical duty to help future patients. She wanted the lawsuit to prevent the pulmonologist, Dr. Peterson, as well as the hematologist, Dr. Mueller, from ever practicing medicine again. She wanted to put a stop to their ability to harm patients. To do so, she wanted every single person involved in Jay's care to provide sworn testimony (deposition) so that her lawyer could demonstrate the pervasive disregard in the face of Jay's worsening condition and Tara's drumbeat of warnings.

But that's not what happened. Tara quickly learned that the legal system, just like the medical system, is guided largely by money. Each deposition costs money, and so the cost would have to be justified with respect to the possible payout at the end. Her lawyer had to pay all the deposition fees and expenses in advance, and if they didn't win the case, he wouldn't be able to recoup those costs. Likewise, expanding the scope to take down the two physicians (as opposed to just settling the case over Jay's death) would increase the cost of the case but wouldn't increase the payout. Therefore, getting the doctors' medical licenses revoked would not be a stated goal of the case.

"Each legal move," Tara said, "felt like it had more to do with the lawyer earning money than it had to do with seeking justice for my husband." It felt eerily similar to her experience as a Clinician Nurse Educator, in which the hospital administrators seemed more concerned about financial liability than about the health of the patient and prevention of future error.

Tara attended the deposition of every physician. "In my idealistic mind," she said, "I assumed that everyone would speak the truth." In her clinical experience, even doctors who were nasty or nurses who were rude still maintained a basic adherence to medical facts. But that was not quite how things played out at the depositions. She expected that Dr. Peterson might fall back on the convenient murkiness of diagnostic uncertainty or conflicting clinical judgments. Or maybe he would say he just couldn't remember. Who could argue with that? But he openly stated things that were in direct conflict with what Tara had observed at Jay's bedside. Dr. Peterson recounted his visit to Jay on what turned out to be Jay's last day alive. He reported that Jay was clinically stable at 1 p.m., and that he and the patient had a "full and easy conversation."

Tara remembered that day all too well. She'd spent the entirety of that day at the bedside watching Jay struggle for air. He could hardly stitch two words together, much less participate in a full and easy conversation. Dr. Peterson further stated in the deposition that no one had alerted him to the patient's decline over the course of the afternoon. The only time he answered, "I don't recall" was when he was asked about Tara's repeated requests for Jay to move to the ICU and her frantic urgings to ramp up the level of care.

Tara was shocked not just at the untruths that Dr. Peterson offered, but at the ease and conviction with which he did so. But from the perspective of the legal system, it was just Tara's word against Dr. Peterson's. It would be left to a jury to decide who sounded more believable, since the only other witness who could have corroborated what did or did not transpire, of course, was Jay.

For Tara, the sense of betrayal cut even deeper when it came to the nurses. *Nurses!* The hospital infantry dedicated to faithful documentation—sometimes to a fault—how could nurses be untruthful under oath? And yet she heard them say things, with a straight face, that strained credulity.

One nurse, for example, had rewritten all eight notes she'd documented over the course of her twelve-hour shift. Rewriting even a single note after the fact is unusual. Rewriting *eight* notes raises a red flag. When questioned about that highly unusual behavior, the nurse said she'd inadvertently written the wrong time and date and so thought it better to rewrite every note in its entirety rather than just correct the time and date.

Tara was dumbfounded. First of all, every nurse knows that if you've written a time or date or really anything in error, the correct course of action is to cross out only the wrong information—though leave it legible—and then write in the correct information immediately adjacent, along with your initials. This indicates that you've noted your error and corrected it. Leaving the original error legible beneath the cross-out shows that you have nothing to hide.

Second, could any nurse make the same error *eight different times* during her shift? By the time you've finished a twelve-hour shift documenting every vital sign and every organ system on every patient on your ward, you may not remember your own name or when you last went to the bathroom, but the one thing you *do* know is the date.

Another nurse denied saying that Jay's gray and mottled skin was a side effect of chemotherapy. For this one, though, a family friend had been present, so Tara knew she had someone to back up her recollection. Still, it was staggering for her to witness her fellow nurses saying things—under oath, no less—that were simply untrue.

The process of depositions and mediation took a grueling three years. There were exhausting negotiations plus endless documents and statements to review. And every step of the way entailed reliving the horrific details of Jay's death. On top of that, Tara had to reconcile how much or how little to share with her children. "In one breath I was telling them their dad died professing his love for them," she said, "and then in another I was seething about the harsh realities of his demise." Sasha and Chris began to avoid talking to her about Jay and grew distant. "But I couldn't contain myself," Tara said, because the details and emotions from the lawsuit seeped into every waking moment of her life. The only way she could prevent herself from inflicting more pain on her children was to simply stop talking. "There were times where I simply didn't speak to them at all," she said.

Throughout this period, the hospital made several financial offers to Tara, offers that came with money but without any admission of wrongdoing. Settling out of court would bring a quick end to the pain of this ordeal. It would also provide immediate financial relief for Tara, who was still struggling to pay off the medical bills. Most important, it would save her from the risk of going to trial and potentially losing the case, and with it, any possibility of a settlement. Tara couldn't ignore the financial reality of a lifetime of raising two children as a single parent, without Jay's help and without the income from his job. Their savings were modest, the bills were considerable, and she was no longer confident of her ability to work as a nurse. A financial settlement could go a long way toward relieving this uncertainty.

But the lies and the evasions Tara heard coming from her professional peers during the depositions disgusted her. "I didn't get the feeling, individually or collectively, that anyone was owning up to their mistakes and poor clinical decisions," she said. Jay was such a straight shooter when it came to taking responsibility for shortcomings, even for the littlest things. She couldn't imagine him standing for the lily-livered equivocations that the medical staff were putting forth. "I didn't believe they acknowledged the systemic problems at their hospital," she said. As a nurse, she could not bring herself to take the settlement without seeing things set right. "I wanted these issues addressed," she said.

Tara turned down the offers. Her lawyer supported her, feeling that she'd have a good chance of winning the case in court. The fact that the hospital kept raising the amount of its offer suggested that it was nervous. After all, the patient had died. Juries tended to be sympathetic in the face of a tragic death.

But if the deposition process had been painful, the preparation for the trial was downright caustic. A week before jury selection, Tara's legal team staged a mock trial so that Tara could become familiar with the proceedings. Tara sat in the witness stand of a pretend courtroom set up at the law firm. Lawyers fired questions at her, and she was instructed to direct her answers toward the jury—in this case a mural of a jury posted on the opposite wall. Tara tried her best to talk to the wall, but it felt awkward and unnatural. She kept instinctively turning back toward the lawyer who was questioning her. Worse, though, she stumbled over her answers. She flubbed easy questions and drew blanks on things she knew well.

At one point the lawyer asked her to relay the words Jay had said to her the night before he died. It was three simple words. Three agonizing words. Three anguishing words that still, to this day, haunt her: "I . . . can't . . . breathe . . ."

Yet at that moment, in the simulated witness stand, she couldn't remember them. Tara frantically turned her mind upside down, trying to recall the three words that had been seared into the membranes of her soul. She became distraught as it grew clear that she wouldn't be able to pull that quote from her memory.

The lawyers observed this panic and so switched to simpler, more mundane questions. They pitched her easy questions about time and place, but still she couldn't come up with answers, even for basic facts. It was hopeless. The legal team finally called off the session. Tara staggered to her feet and could hardly keep herself upright as she tottered toward the door.

Five days later—the day before jury selection—the hospital increased its offer significantly. By this time, Tara was nauseated and shaky almost every day, hardly eating or sleeping. Her weight, which had recovered in the prior year, dropped back down to ninety pounds. "I felt paralyzed," she said, "as if something was strangling me. I didn't believe I could survive the trial. I knew my kids would be present, and they would have to observe me falling apart. I finally realized that I couldn't save this hospital's broken system any more than I was able to save Jay." She accepted the settlement, even though the hospital would not admit any wrongdoing.

---

Receiving money after the loss of a loved one is discordant by any human logic. Trying to replace the irreplaceable is already an impossibility, excruciating even to contemplate. Filling that hole with the crassest of commodities can seem like an insult to the human spirit. And yet . . .

And yet, that is what we do in our legal system to redress medical errors. That is what Tara received after losing the love of her life—a check. It seems almost horrifying to contemplate these two concepts in a single sentence—a beloved human being and a piece of paper with numbers on it.

A supreme unfairness. And yet . . .

And yet, money can make a tangible difference. Besides the bills that needed to be paid, Tara discovered that the practical parts of recovery were expensive. Therapy wasn't cheap—or easy—but it enabled Tara and her children to grapple with the trauma from Jay's sudden and violent absence from their lives. It took years of therapy for Tara to deescalate the paralyzing flashbacks of witnessing Jay's death. The money also enabled her to visit her children when they left for college, to help them with the painful emotions that trailed them for years.

But the money didn't restore Tara's faith in the medical system. It didn't repair the strained relationships with family and friends. It didn't bring back the years lost to suffering and grief. And, of course, it didn't bring back Jay. It didn't create a father for Sasha and Chris. It didn't fill the throbbing, bottomless hole created by the loss of a life partner. It just made an awful experience a few degrees less awful.

Tara fully recognized how much worse life would have been *without* the financial settlement. Experiencing grief, PTSD, and insomnia while simultaneously trying to exude strength and solidity for her children, who were experiencing crushing emotional devastation of their own, was hard enough. To do that while sinking financially would have been unspeakably cruel, though that is a fate that many people face.

---

Malpractice suits are far from perfect. Because of the cost, effort, and stringency involved, they are available only to a tiny fraction of patients who've experienced medical error. Additionally, there is little consistency within malpractice law: different juries can come to opposite conclusions on similar sets of facts, and payouts for patients vary tremendously. Beyond this, there is the side effect of defensive medicine—all the additional testing and treatment that doctors undertake because of the fear of lawsuits, whether real or imagined.

In addition to estimated costs of $45–55 billion wasted on defensive medicine, there is the actual harm that can come from this unnecessary treatment. Just the superfluous CT scans alone can lead to kidney damage from IV contrast, additional cancers from the extra radiation, and, of course, false positive diagnoses from the plethora of incidental findings that pop up like mushrooms after a spring rain.

Given all of these drawbacks, it's reasonable to ask whether lawsuits actually work. Does the malpractice system make medicine safer? This is tough to answer with any reliability because you can't really do a randomized controlled trial. Researchers who've examined the data estimate that only about 7% of patients who've been harmed by negligent medical care ever receive any compensation. On the flip side, fewer than 20% of people who receive compensation actually suffered from negligent care. Additionally, more than half the money paid out goes to cover litigation costs rather than to the patients themselves. So at the very least, it is an inefficient system.[2] Many in the medical community believe that rather than improving patient safety, the system simply causes doctors to practice defensive medicine.

Most malpractice lawyers, perhaps unsurprisingly, say the malpractice system is beneficial to patient safety. "The fact is," Seattle-based lawyer Peter Mullenix told me, "the medical profession does not do a very good job of policing itself." A malpractice case speaks not only to the doctors who have acted carelessly, "but also to all of the other doctors who know that doctor." There is a ripple effect across the medical community that affects both individual practitioners and regulatory boards, imbuing these lawsuits with a powerful potential to save lives. "For every malpractice case," Mullenix said, "there are probably fifteen doctors who look at it and say, 'I'd better not do that!'" He made the analogy to car safety: "We now have seatbelts, airbags, and excellent brakes because the system held the automotive industry liable."

You will surely not be surprised that most doctors beg to differ on this viewpoint. Certainly most British doctors did not react that way after Hadiza Bawa-Garba was convicted of manslaughter in the death of young Jack Adcock. The general sentiment was more along the anguished lines of "There but for the grace of God go I." They saw a scenario that they'd all been in— overworked, understaffed, dealing with malfunctioning technology, perhaps cutting a few corners in order to survive an impossible workload. Rather than learning lessons about medical actions they shouldn't do, they saw the court as a weapon to scapegoat doctors for the shortcomings of the entire medical system.

But even beyond that extreme case in which there was a highly unusual criminal conviction, the threat of a lawsuit—even in theory—strikes fear in the hearts of most doctors. Even knowing that doctors win most cases doesn't assuage the terror or reduce the aggressive over-testing and overtreatment from defensive medicine. Sara Charles, a psychiatrist I interviewed for an earlier book, *What Doctors Feel*, described to me a bruising lawsuit that is emblematic of many doctors' experiences. A patient of Sara's attempted suicide by jumping off a rooftop. The patient survived, though she was permanently injured, and sued Sara for negligence in her care. The patient contended that Sara did not appropriately treat her depression and that this negligence resulted in her suicidality and severe injury.

Sara ultimately "won" the case, but even she would put that word in quotation marks. The fact that the jury found that she had not been negligent could hardly make up for the five agonizing years Sara suffered. Her personal and professional lives were ravaged by the experience, and being vindicated hardly offered relief. When Sara began to research malpractice, she realized that her experiences were depressingly common among physicians. Moreover, her patient ultimately wasn't helped by the experience either. It was the same five miserable years for her, with nothing at the end to make it worthwhile. The lawsuit didn't improve the patient's situation and it didn't make Sara a better doctor. The only change to Sara's practice was that she became hesitant to take on patients with more severe psychiatric conditions.

While some errors are committed by medical personnel who are truly negligent and substandard, the vast majority of errors are committed unintentionally by otherwise conscientious doctors and nurses. For these folks, malpractice suits do not serve to educate or improve. The devastating outcome for their patients usually delivers a powerful enough dose of grief, shame, and awareness of the error. There is rarely much constructive gain that malpractice suits can add to individuals who recognize their errors and feel remorse about them. Many, like Sara, shy away from complicated patients after that, thus decreasing medical options for very sick patients. In a survey of four thousand doctors, more than half who'd been sued reported that malpractice fears influenced their care with every or nearly every patient. Even the doctors who had *never* been sued felt that way—40% reported the same behavior.[3]

Doctors who've been sued commonly experience depression, anxiety, isolation, and loss of trust in the doctor-patient relationship. The effect can be so shattering that the term "clinical judicial syndrome" has been developed to encompass the depth and breadth of the fallout.[4] Though it never denies the primacy of the damage to the "first victim" (the patient), clinical judicial syndrome recognizes that medical error can also create a "second victim." Doctors often experience their personal and professional lives being shredded during a very public and humiliating process, one that can drag on for years. Many have likened the emotional trauma to experiencing a death in the family, and some never recover. While the general public, perhaps understandably, might be loath to yank out the violin for well-paid doctors, it's important to note that up to 40% of lawsuits turn out to contain no medical error at all.[5]

A not-insubstantial number of doctors, therefore, have their lives upended when they haven't done anything wrong.

Peter Mullenix has a different take on this. "The weird thing about malpractice," he said, "is that doctors, unlike any other profession, seem to think they should be immune from consequences of their carelessness because their ultimate goal is to help people." He points out that altruism exists in many other lines of work. Architects, engineers, lawyers, and plumbers are all trying to help people. "Every profession has members who make careless choices that sometimes harm people. But it only seems to be doctors who think the law should protect them against their bad choices because their motivation is to help people. If a lawyer commits malpractice, the lawyer expects to face legal consequences. But doctors don't think it's fair and they've been able to set the system up to avoid accountability in all but the most egregious cases."

When it comes to institutions—as opposed to individuals—there seems to be evidence that direct legal action and financial penalties can be effective. For example, when Medicare starting fining hospitals for high rates of certain complications that were felt to be avoidable—bed sores, falls, blood clots, hospital-acquired infections—hospitals moved quickly to clean up their act. As with the auto industry, the bottom line is a powerful motivator.

The bottom line, however, isn't always effective for individuals. For most doctors and nurses—as opposed to institutions—money is, at best, an oblique incentive. We all want our patients to do well. No clinician with a detectible heartbeat wants her patient to get a hospital-acquired infection, or have surgery on the wrong side of the body, or receive a delayed diagnosis of cancer. Threats of lawsuits are not necessary to instill this priority.

The adversarial nature of litigation also runs counter to the general mode of medical learning, which involves gradual accrual of evidence leading toward a consensus. Doctors and nurses generally see themselves as being on the same side as the patient, wanting things to work better. Committed clinicians expect to be held accountable when they fall short, but adversarial litigation usually ends up embittering rather than engaging. We'd much rather an adverse outcome rally doctors and nurses to improve the system, not cause them to sequester themselves behind a wall of defensive medicine.

For cases of blatant medical negligence or egregious medical care, litigation is clearly appropriate. But for most adverse outcomes and for errors that are not a result of callous disregard, the malpractice system is an unwieldy tool. From the patient perspective, it is inefficient because it can aid only those for whom vast financial damages can be calculated. If the potential recoverable amount doesn't exceed the prodigious cost of litigation, it's not worth the patient's or the lawyer's time, so nothing happens.

Peter Mullenix, the malpractice attorney, told me he has to turn down 99% of cases that come to his firm, either because it's not possible to prove causality or because the damages are not extensive enough to merit the costs. He estimates his firm has to spend up to $200,000 per case, so he needs to be sure the ultimate payout will cover this. They have to hire experts on standard-of-care for the medical issue at hand, experts knowledgeable about medical records, and experts on the calculation of damages. Sometimes law firms have to hire economists and experts on government regulations. They have to conduct depositions of witnesses for both the prosecution and the defense. The witnesses and experts can be scattered geographically, so travel expenses figure in.

In light of this, they will only take a case that seems winnable, in which the doctor's liability is obvious and egregious, such as ignoring a clear-cut infection or misdiagnosing an evident cancer. To generate a potential settlement that will cover all the costs, plus the lawyers' fees, plus a worthwhile payout for the patient, means the firm can only take a case in which calculated damages are severe—medical bills in the millions, a patient who is left permanently paralyzed or requires lifelong care or has died.

Only about 1% of cases that come to their firm fit these criteria.

Mullenix said he found it saddening that so many patients—even those who experienced legitimate errors—weren't able to muster a winnable case. It was painful to explain, over and over, that even if you suffered harm or had a bad outcome, the malpractice system wouldn't be able to help you. His frustration with the narrow reach of his professional world led him to the arena of patient-safety advocacy.

Mullenix joined the Washington Advocates for Patient Safety as a way to help patients for whom the malpractice system is inadequate. The goal of WAPS is to help minimize medical errors and patient harm. This involves working on legislation, raising awareness, educating medical professionals, educating patients and families, and providing resources. Mullenix's particular interest resides in the area of medical devices—artificial joints, pacemakers, surgical tools, and the like. He'd been shocked to learn how lightly medical devices are regulated and how sales representatives are often present in the operating room alongside the surgeons.

Patient-safety advocates, as I'll discuss in chapter 13, have become another rung of scaffolding in the effort to decrease medical error. Most enter the arena the hard way, after struggling through a wrenching and often isolating medical experience. Typically patient-safety advocates find each other online or by word of mouth, with battle-weary recognition of kindred spirits. Even for the rare few who have been vindicated and won a lawsuit, the trauma remains. As Tara learned, the money may help with the overwhelming bills, but it never makes up for the lost loved one or any of the permanent damage suffered. And it certainly doesn't fix the system.

---

"The system in which Jay died was undeniably broken," Tara reflected, "partly because of an atmosphere of secrecy. The nurses could not admit to what they didn't know. And, I suspect, neither could the doctors. Dr. Peterson prided himself on his twenty-plus years of doctordom. I got the feeling he used that line a lot: 'In my twenty-plus years of experience, blah, blah, blah.' He seemed like the type of doctor who'd be dismissive of anyone with less polished credentials, a guy who'd intimidate those around him from questioning his judgment."

When the hospital offered to settle out of court, Tara wanted a commitment from it to improve the conditions she felt had led to Jay's death. She wanted them to confront the shoddy communication among the staff. She wanted them to lower the barriers to transferring patients to the ICU. She wanted the hospital to mandate nursing education about sepsis. She wanted hospital leadership to commit to engaging patients and families in a meaningful way.

What was the hospital's response? It offered to put up a plaque in the BMTU in memory of Jay. Tara could hardly contain her rage. A plaque?!? At her creative best, Tara could not have come up with a more apt metaphor for the hospital's myopia—nailing a piece of wood on a wall instead of training the staff about sepsis, critical care, and communication.

The hospital came back with an offer to hold an annual lecture in Jay's name. This piqued Tara's interest, as it might actually translate to education and improved patient care. But it turned out that the lecture would only be for the medical students, not the BMTU staff. And when Tara asked if she could be one of the speakers, the hospital flatly refused.

In desperation, Tara requested a single meeting with the BMTU staff, a roundtable discussion where, at the very least, they could review the case and the lessons learned. At first glance this sounds like the least desirable thing to request in a settlement: an intimate engagement with the people you felt had killed your husband. But at some point, almost all patients and family members facing medical error find they are simply too exhausted for revenge. It's too painful and too depleting and, ultimately, fruitless. The error will not unwind. Your loved one will not walk in the door. The damage will not reverse.

Tara had been run ragged by the three-year legal process and her own grief, as well as that of her two children. The only meager light anywhere in that endless tunnel was the chance to protect future patients from what Jay had experienced. A face-to-face meeting with the BMTU staff was about the only thing she could effect at this point. The hospital agreed.

Tara channeled whatever energy she had left into this roundtable discussion. She prepared relentlessly for the meeting, spending months organizing documents and handouts, rehearsing what she would say. She didn't want to alienate the staff; she wanted to engage them as a colleague from the medical trenches. She understood their world—she wanted them to know that—but she needed them to understand hers. She wanted to impress upon the staff the human dimensions of their actions and how to prevent a future error.

The roundtable meeting was held in a hospital conference room. Tara scanned the staff as they filed in—not one of the doctors was there. Not one of the floor nurses from the BMTU was there. The only people Tara recognized were Constance—the nurse manager of the BMTU who was more of an administrator—and the hospital's attorney. Tara knew that Dr. Everett had moved to a new hospital and that the two hematology fellows—Dr. Samir and Dr. Chowdury—had graduated by this time, but Dr. Mueller and Dr. Peterson were still on staff. The attending hematologist and pulmonologist were the two doctors most responsible for the decision-making in Jay's case. Where were they? And the floor nurses who performed the daily care for Jay, who were the ones that Tara reported her observations to—where were they? Their absence stung.

This wasn't what Tara had in mind when she'd requested the meeting. She wanted to have a direct discussion with the clinical staff, the ones actually taking care of patients. The ones who'd taken care of Jay. Instead, she faced ten administrators and nurse managers who looked as though they'd been frog-marched in at gunpoint.

She had no choice, though, but to plow forward. Tara opened the meeting by passing out photos of Jay. She wanted to them to see the person he was—father, husband, friend, aviator. But the atmosphere around the table was cold. Nobody spoke or made much of any connection. The discussion that Tara had hoped for turned into a monologue, but she persevered, describing Jay and what had transpired during his one-hundred-hour stay in the BMTU. Tara distributed copies of the state's nursing code of ethics, sliding the sheets along the leaden chill of the vast oak table.

Would these words even mean anything? she wondered. Would these nurses-turned-bureaucrats even remember what it was like to look into the eyes of a terrified, critically ill patient? Or were they too far gone? Too sunk in their monthly reports to recall the feel of a racing pulse beneath fevered skin. Too enmeshed in their policy manuals to remember the give of a syringe or the bristle of gauze. Did they still retain the instinct of how to transfer a patient from gurney to bed without unsettling IVs, catheters, or a patient's trust? Could their hand muscles even summon up the brisk squeezes to inflate a blood pressure cuff?

Tara told them that she well understood the severity of AML and that she'd harbored no illusions about Jay's prognosis. She knew from her own nursing experience that MRSA sepsis was ferocious. She knew that Jay might have died even if his sepsis had been treated appropriately. But it hadn't been—and that was why she was in this conference room right now.

If Jay had been intubated when he could no longer breathe and been transferred to the ICU when his condition grew critical, she would have understood his death. She would have accepted Jay's death as a tragic outcome of a terrible disease complicated by a virulent infection. But that's not what happened. "No one paid attention to the signs and symptoms of sepsis he was exhibiting," she told them. That by itself was substandard medicine. But even if the staff didn't notice Jay's worsening condition, there was Tara—the patient's wife, yes, but also a trained RN—pointing it out to them over and over. "No one listened to my concerns," she said to the group.

As a result, Jay was never offered the high-intensity care of the ICU that would have given his body a fighting chance of eradicating the MRSA infection. He might not have survived even in the ICU, true, but there was a chance that he might have. And if he pulled through the sepsis, then the AML treatment could continue with the goal of a bone marrow transplant, which was Jay's only chance for a cure. Tara knew that the bone marrow transplant held its own grave risks, and that the odds of a cure were long—but they weren't zero. And if you are thirty-nine years old and have two children, you deserve that chance, however slim. But by ignoring the signs of worsening sepsis, the BMTU staff deprived Jay—and deprived his children—of that singular chance.

Tara talked about the importance of training nurses on the BMTU about sepsis, since their patients were at especially high risk. She also talked about the nurses' role in educating family members about noticing—and reporting—any concerning signs. Tara had learned, after the fact, that family members themselves were allowed to initiate a "rapid response" that would call an emergency team to the bedside. Had she known that, she would have done so, but the nurses had never told her. She stressed how critical it was for the nurses to inform patients and their families about that option.

Tara's audience sat in rigid silence. Nobody moved. Nobody spoke. There wasn't the slightest twitch from the 430 collective facial muscles gathered grimly around the table. If there had been cardiac monitors in the room, they would have registered a collective flat line. But Tara pressed on. "I wasn't nervous at all," she recalled. "This felt right, and I felt Jay's energy all around me."

Tara told the group about the profound guilt she was saddled with: she—an experienced ER and CCU nurse—had allowed Jay to die on her watch. She could never forgive herself for that. She described to them her predicament at the bedside, trying to navigate her role as the supportive spouse versus that of the instinctive nurse. At that moment, a solitary whimper escaped from her. It echoed in the room against the rigid surfaces and silent bodies. Tara quickly corralled her composure; she was not going to break down in front of these people and be dismissed as the overemotional wife.

She pleaded for them to learn from Jay's death, imploring them to spend more time and money educating the nursing staff. Tara explained that she hadn't wanted to sue—that was neither her nature nor her philosophy. Litigation against her own profession was downright devastating. She'd finally brought the suit only because she'd learned that hospitals attend to problems only when major dollars are at stake.

But she felt as if her words were evaporating into the walls that were painted corporate-compliance gray. Everyone at the table appeared to be watching the second hand on the clock, counting down the time until they could get back to their spreadsheets and quarterly reports. Tara was about to wrap up the meeting when Constance, the nurse manager of the BMTU, asked if she could speak.

"I remember Jay," Constance said quietly, "and so do others from the floor. He has not been forgotten." Tears began to well up in her eyes, and Tara felt her own heart ache. Maybe, Tara thought, I haven't been the only one suffering with guilt.

"What happened was horrible," Constance said, as the hospital's lawyer squirmed visibly in his chair. "That day was the worst day of my medical career," Constance continued, ignoring him, "and I am deeply sorry for what happened."

Then she looked directly at Tara and said, "You tried harder than anyone to save Jay."

It was almost audible, the first faint splintering of Tara's strangling guilt. Somebody—*somebody*—recognized her efforts. Constance's words offered the first stuttering glimmers of reprieve. Maybe Tara *wasn't* the worthless nurse she'd been feeling like, or the useless wife, or the feckless advocate. Maybe Jay *didn't* die because she wasn't smart enough, or tenacious enough, or dedicated enough. Maybe, just maybe, Jay's death wasn't her fault.

Tara had been determined not to cry during this meeting—nothing would get her written off more efficiently than a puddle of tears—but she could hold back no longer. It was clear that there would be no resolution with any of the doctors. And no resolution with any of the floor nurses who had been caring for Jay. "Thank you," she choked out to Constance. "Thank you for saving my life." This single exchange with the nurse manager would be the only human response Tara would ever get from the hospital system.

# CHAPTER TWELVE

# IS THERE A BETTER WAY?

If the American malpractice system is so arduous and expensive and is unavailable to the vast majority of patients who've experienced errors, it's fair to ask whether there might be a better way. How do other countries handle medical error?

Whether it's self-assembled furniture, aerodynamically soled shoes, prison reform, recycling, saunas, or just plain old happiness, Scandinavia strikes many as the land of the sensible. So perhaps it's no accident that some of the most thoughtful ideas about handling medical error originate from the latitudes that require industrial-strength thermal underwear.

Denmark is an intriguing case study, because although it has the polar opposite system of healthcare coverage (national health insurance versus the largely private US system), it actually started with a similar malpractice system, although on a far smaller scale. Prior to 1992, patients who felt they'd been harmed in the medical system had to take their case to court. They faced the same hurdles that American patients face—tough to get the case litigated if damages weren't financially compelling enough and even tougher to prove actual negligence. In practice, the majority of patients who'd experienced error had no recourse.

In 1992, the country decided to fall in line with its Nordic neighbors and adopt a no-fault compensation system.[1] The idea of this system is to award a modest compensation to any patient whose care wasn't as good as it should have been or to any patient who experienced a rare or severe complication. Whether the bad outcome happened because of an error or because of negligence or from plain-old bad luck is irrelevant.

By eliminating the burden of proving negligence, far more patients can benefit. And by taking out the adversarial component, doctors aren't on the defensive. This Patient Compensation System, as it came to be called in Denmark, eliminated the major hurdles that patients faced in the old malpractice court system. It's much easier to access because you don't have to find a lawyer willing to take your case. It's also simpler, because there's only one sheet of paper to fill out. It's also free, so there's no financial barrier to patients. Doctors and hospitals can even file on behalf of patients, and often do.

The cases are adjudicated by an administrative panel similar to the American workers' compensation board. The panel is made up of legal and medical experts who review the details of the patient's case, along with a response from the doctor or hospital involved. The patient is awarded compensation if the medical care is deemed to have been substandard (compared to the standard-of-care from a highly trained professional in that field) or if the poor outcome is considered "more extensive than a patient should reasonably have to endure."[2] Typically, about one-third of the cases are deemed worthy of compensation. There is an appeals process for patients who are turned down, though very few patients go that route.

Because patients don't face the daunting burden of proving negligence, a much higher percentage of injured patients in Denmark receive financial compensation (about four times as many as American patients, when adjusted for population size). Danish patients usually receive payment within seven or eight months, compared to an average of five years for American patients who file lawsuits.

The payouts are quite modest by American standards—$30,000 on average—but monumental settlements aren't necessary because nationalized healthcare ensures that Danes never face the mountains of medical bills that Americans do. And even for patients whose cases don't prevail—or for patients who don't bother filing a claim—most Danes won't be bankrupted by their injuries because social services are more readily available. Unemployment and disability benefits, in particular, are generous. All Danes receive a pension after retirement. They don't accrue debt from big-ticket items such as daycare and college, since those are all free. And of course Danes, unlike Americans, never worry about losing health insurance if they lose their jobs because healthcare is guaranteed for all.

You might not be surprised to learn that Denmark ranks as one of the happiest countries in the world. They invented Legos, after all, and boast the world's oldest amusement park—in operation since 1583. But if you are booking your tickets to Copenhagen as we speak, just remember that in the dead of winter, the sun sets by early afternoon. And there's always Kierkegaard or *Hamlet* to put you in a gloomy mood.

———————————

In the summer of 1997, a few years after the Patient Compensation System debuted, Dr. Beth Lilja and her family took a vacation in Carriacou. For a busy obstetrician, a remote island in the Caribbean seemed an ideal place to unwind—nothing but pristine beach in its twelve square miles of territory. But remoteness has its downsides. When Lilja exhausted her reading material, she learned that there weren't any bookstores on the island where she could restock. So when her colleague arrived from New York to join her on the vacation, she quickly pounced on the bulging Sunday edition of the *New York Times* that he'd thoughtfully stowed in his carry-on.

The cover story of the magazine section immediately caught her eye with the arresting title: "How Can We Save the Next Victim?"[3] The article profiled two-month-old Jose Martinez, a baby with a congenital heart defect who was treated with intravenous digoxin for the symptoms of congestive heart failure. Digoxin, originally extracted from the bell-shaped foxglove flower, has an exceedingly narrow safety margin—meaning that there is not much daylight between treatment doses and toxic doses. (Among the side effects of digoxin—besides nausea, vomiting, cardiac arrhythmias, and death—are seeing unusual yellow-green halos. Some historians believe that van Gogh was taking foxglove—he'd painted his own physician holding the flower—and that this side effect might have been responsible for the striking yellow swirls in *The Starry Night*.)

Because of the narrow safety margin—especially in children—the dose of digoxin is based on weight, calculated as milligrams per kilogram. The resident and the attending taking care of Jose did the calculations together and came up with the correct dose of 0.09 milligrams. The resident then wrote the medication orders in the chart but inadvertently moved the decimal point and wrote 0.9 milligrams instead of 0.09 milligrams. Baby Jose died from receiving a dose of digoxin that was ten-fold too high.

Lilja found herself both horrified and engrossed. It was like an opera where you know the tragic ending in advance but can't stop the characters from blundering down the fatal pathway. The article ran through all the steps in minute detail, steps that were meant to provide protection but consistently malfunctioned. The attending, for example, was required to review the resident's orders as part of the standard oversight, which he did. But his eyes didn't catch the subtle decimal-shift error. A pharmacist who was concerned about the dose paged the resident, but had no way of knowing that the resident had left for the day. A backup order was later received by a pharmacy technician who didn't know about the other pharmacist's hesitation and so filled the order. The nurse who received the medication was concerned about the dose and so appropriately asked a covering resident to recheck the calculation. The resident redid the formula on his calculator, but when looking from the calculator with the correct answer of 0.09 milligrams to the vial of 0.9 milligrams didn't notice the decimal difference. As a last check, the concerned nurse asked a second nurse to recheck the vial and compare it to the order; the second nurse saw 0.9 on both and confirmed that this was correct. The fatal dose was administered.

What especially fascinated Lilja was that the analysis focused on the problems of the system rather than the incompetence or negligence of the medical staff. In fact the staff seemed quite conscientious, putting in extra efforts at every step of the way in attempt to avoid error. Yet the incorrect dose nevertheless barreled its way through all the layers of protection, just as Bob Wachter witnessed two decades later when Pablo Garcia received 38½ tablets of Bactrim.

In Denmark, the general perception of the medical field was that the practice of medicine was basically safe, apart from the occasional mistakes of individuals. Even though the new Patient Compensation System did not focus on finding fault, the emphasis was still on identifying the bad apples and helping them mend their erroneous ways. This was the first time Lilja had read of researchers explicitly strategizing about how to make the system safer for the next patient, not which doctors or nurses to fire.

Lilja packed the article along with her sunscreen and took it back to Denmark with her. As it happened, she was embarking on a new job as a senior obstetrician, and would shortly be facing the obligatory meeting with the medical director, who would be asking the obligatory question about her research interests. Now she had a ready answer.

---

For decades, the *British Medical Journal*, or *BMJ*, had always graced its covers with the weekly table of contents. High art it wasn't, but it served its purpose. Medical journals aren't elbowing for space with *Cosmopolitan* and *People* on grocery store magazine stands. They don't need surgically sculpted movie stars or sordid infidelity headlines to entice readers to pick them up. The fixed readership of doctors and researchers are generally simple folk in this regard: they just need to know which studies they have to be up on and which page to turn to. A dutiful list of articles on a utilitarian blue background has long sufficed.

But on March 18, 2000, the *BMJ* ditched its reserved presentation and covered its journal with a picture of a plane crash. It was an issue devoted to patient safety, inspired by the 1999 report *To Err Is Human* from the Institute of Medicine in the US. (The medical-error-as-third-leading-cause-of-death article came sixteen years later in the very same *BMJ*.) The media had been having a field day with jumbo jet metaphors for medical error ever since Lucian Leape coined that analogy in 1994. For this special issue on patient safety, the *BMJ* borrowed that riveting imagery. Its other not-so-subliminal message was that medicine should learn from the aviation industry's efforts to understand and reduce plane crashes.

Beth Lilja remembers the issue vividly and read it cover to cover. Every article was focused on fixing the system, not just reeducating the bad apples. It coincided with an international conference on patient safety where she got to meet Leape and many of the pioneers of the patient-safety movement.

Inspired by—or rather, horrified by—the IOM estimates that some one hundred thousand Americans died because of medical error each year, Lilja and her colleagues undertook their own study to assess the state of medical error on their home turf. Everyone regarded the Danish medical system as exemplary, with the highest standards of care. But in fact, Lilja's study revealed an error rate comparable to what had been cited by the IOM. Her report was set to upend the status quo in Denmark, just as *To Err Is Human* had done in the US. But as events turned out, the report was published on the morning of September 11, 2001.

Because of the time difference, the 9/11 terrorist attacks in the United States did not make the front page of the Danish newspapers until September 12. So on September 11, the Danish medical-error study was on the front page, but it was quickly buried. Lilja was scheduled for a TV interview the following week, but she remembers being told that her appearance was conditional, "depending if we do or don't have a war."

Lilja was eventually interviewed by the television station, but international terrorism dominated everyone's attention in the weeks and months that followed. "The report didn't get much press," Louise Rabøl, a public health physician, told me, "but this turned out to be an advantage." In the hushed atmosphere following 9/11, the nascent patient-safety community in Denmark was able to sift through the report without much interference from politicians or the press. The somberness of the international mood combined with the innate pragmatism of Danes led to a sober search for solutions without any grandstanding or petty grievances. It just didn't feel seemly.

The report slowly gained traction in the medical community. For Danes who are used to being applauded for their efficient solutions to nearly every societal ill, the recognition of a high medical-error rate "was a real wakeup call," according to Rabøl. Within a few months, the main stakeholders in the healthcare system created the Danish Society for Patient Safety, which included representatives from every group with skin in the game—doctors, nurses, midwives, hospitals, research institutions, patient organizations, pharmacies, and drug companies. Away from the geopolitical tumult of the day, the group began to draw up a framework to address medical error by seeking to improve the system as a whole.

Being largely ignored by the preoccupied outside world allowed the various parties to work together with less than the usual friction. Their goal was to have the medical system be open and transparent about errors, and that no one would be afraid to report adverse events. This reporting would provide a road map for future improvements. But in order to achieve this, there would have to be a law setting out the terms.

When Lilja approached the minister of health with the idea of a Patient Safety Act, he said, "If you can guarantee that no main organization will block it, I'll do it." Lilja set about, as she described it, going door to door, talking to everyone she could find with any vested interest in medical error. Most doctors she spoke to had mixed feelings about owning up publicly to an error. They supported it in theory, but when it came to the actual practice, they were hesitant.

One of Lilja's colleagues—whom she described as "very conservative"—was initially opposed to the idea. But then he related a story to Lilja. One day, when he was a trainee, he was paged to administer an IV antibiotic to a patient. He'd been on his way out the door to go home, but he returned to the ward as instructed. He was told which patient needed the antibiotic and set about injecting the medication. Just as he was reaching the end of the injection, the patient said, almost offhandedly, "You know, I'm allergic to penicillin." The doctor froze, because in his hand sat a nearly empty syringe of penicillin.

The young doctor was too afraid to say anything—to the patient, to the nurses, to his colleagues. Instead, he stayed at the patient's bedside for the next two hours, taking her blood pressure every five minutes so that he might detect the very first signs of an allergic reaction or potentially fatal anaphylaxis. Two hours went by, and nary an itch nor a rash nor a welt emerged. The blood pressure and pulse hadn't budged a wink. Like so many people, she'd probably had a minor side effect with penicillin as a child and been told, incorrectly, that she was allergic. Over the years, this "fact" solidified into her medical history.

The doctor-in-training went home that night, relieved that he hadn't harmed the patient but fraught with discomfort. "I could have told the patient that she actually didn't have an allergy," he said to Lilja. "That would have been valuable information for her." But this would have meant owning up to his error—something that was shameful and uncomfortable. He'd be blamed by his colleagues, even laughed at. He would have to endure the bureaucratic medical-error gauntlet, getting beaten down with blame at every step of the way. It was easier just to keep quiet, especially since no harm had been done.

"That patient probably still thinks she has a penicillin allergy today," he observed ruefully. He knew he'd done a disservice to the patient—what if she needed a penicillin-related antibiotic in the future and ended up using a less effective or more toxic one instead? This thought haunted him for years. His lasting regret over that situation ultimately converted him to Lilja's point of view. Transparency about medical error would ultimately be better for everyone.

When the recommendations for the Patient Safety Act were presented to the public and to politicians, every sector of Danish society interested in patient safety was on board. And when the bill came before Parliament in 2003, the law was passed with a unanimous vote.

The main accomplishment of the Patient Safety Act was the creation of the National Incident Reporting System. Anyone working in healthcare could report any adverse event. The sole goal of this repository of data would be improving the healthcare system; nothing reported to this system could be used for compensation, disciplinary action, complaints, or litigation. The law explicitly stated that doctors could not be sued based on information reported to the Incident Reporting System. "We were very careful with the wording," Lilja said, because doctors wouldn't report adverse events if they thought they'd be incriminating themselves.

If an adverse event is separately reported to the Patient Compensation System—by a patient, for example—then the doctors' actions might be investigated. But anything reported to the Incident Reporting System is legally cordoned off. Incidents can even be reported anonymously, but it's a credit to the trust in the system that this only happens in 3% of reported cases.

"We all go to work trying to do our best," Rabøl observed. "So if something goes wrong, we want to know how we can improve it." The goal of the Incident Reporting System is to encourage all healthcare workers—the ground troops who see what's actually going on—to inform the system of any problems. "For that reason," Rabøl said, "we don't call it *filing* a report. It's just reporting a problem." The law was later extended to allow patients and families to report incidents as well.

These accumulated reports add up to a critical mass of data. Researchers can then identify problem areas and direct efforts toward improvements.

Rabøl cited the example of pressure ulcers (also known as decubitus ulcers). In the past, these ulcers were considered an inevitable outcome in hospitalized patients who were stuck in bed for days or weeks at a time; they weren't even considered adverse events. For most healthcare workers, pressure ulcers were in the same mental category as the black-and-blue marks patients got from IVs and blood draws.

Starting in 2004, medical staff were told not just to report problems but to report *every single thing* that was not part of the intended treatment. Suddenly it seemed as though there was an epidemic of pressure ulcers in Denmark. Of course there was no such epidemic; it was just that now these ulcers were being reported.

Once the scope of the problem became clear, the medical system began an aggressive prevention effort. Within a few years, the ulcer rate plummeted. Now, advanced pressure ulcers (stages 2, 3, and 4) are hardly ever seen in Denmark. Only stage 1 ulcers are seen, and even these have become much less common. "When we pay attention," Rabøl said, "we can eliminate them. But if we take our eyes off them, they come back!"

The whole approach to medical error in Denmark impressed me. It all seemed so level-headed, so reasonable, so downright Danish. "It works because we trust our state," Rabøl said with a laugh. "We don't sue each other. We have a high degree of trust in society. There's very little corruption. We pay our taxes gladly because we know they are used well."

---

Could such a system possibly work in the US? Obviously the stark difference between national healthcare in Denmark and privatized healthcare in the US makes direct translation tricky. Additionally, there is the notable difference in scale: the population of Denmark is just a smidge larger than Brooklyn and Queens put together (5.5 million people) versus the US population of 325 million. And then there is the vast imbalance in the sums of money involved. The US spends almost 18% of its GDP on healthcare, about $3.3 trillion. Denmark, by contrast, spends only 10% of its GDP on healthcare, about $3 billion—less than what Americans collectively spend on dental floss and tattoos.[4]

So is there any possibility that sensible approaches from the land of *hygge* coziness could make it in the Wild West of brash capitalists? The muscular leitmotif of American individualism makes it unlikely that the adversarial legal approach to medical error will recede any time soon. However, there are some small experiments that offer tantalizing possibilities. But none of these arose from Danish-style sober, unanimous, collaborative decision-making.

Rather, these American experiments arose from knife-to-the-jugular public health emergencies.

In the 1970s and '80s the number of malpractice cases and the size of payouts in the United States were rising rapidly—especially for injuries related to childbirth. The cost of insuring obstetricians grew so extravagant that many insurers stopped offering malpractice coverage, especially in Virginia and Florida. In the space of five years, twenty insurance carriers in Florida pulled out, leading to a contagion of price hikes by the remaining carriers. Doctors' premiums quadrupled. In some areas of Florida, obstetricians faced insurance bills that were as much as seven times higher than those of their colleagues in New York or California, and they threatened to close up shop. A growing sense of crisis ensued, with the looming specter—fed perhaps by an overzealous media—of women in labor being turned away from hospitals, left to deliver babies on the sidewalk with hapless taxi drivers assuming the bulk of obstetrical care.

The state legislatures had no choice but to intervene. They decided to focus on the high-profile birth injuries that cause neurological damage, injuries loosely gathered under the umbrella term of cerebral palsy. Traditionally, cerebral palsy was thought to be due entirely to lack of oxygen to the baby during delivery (i.e., it was the fault of the doctor) but newer research suggested an array of complex factors including genetics, environmental exposures, and interrelated medical conditions. The difficulty in sorting out the causal factors made these cases particularly expensive to pursue, with extensive pretrial research and swarms of expert witnesses. Moreover, the need for intensive, long-term medical care for these infants resulted in exorbitant payouts. This combination made these lawsuits singularly expensive to litigate, resulting in a snowball effect on the whole medical ecosystem.

Toward the end of the 1980s, Virginia and Florida set up state-run compensation funds for birth-related neurological injuries. The thinking was that if this chunk of costly cases was pulled out of the courts, then the malpractice system for everything else would stabilize. Insurance premiums for doctors would level out, doctors wouldn't retire in droves, and taxi drivers could focus on changing lanes without signaling rather than tying off umbilical cords with jumper cables.

On the federal level, the National Vaccine Injury Compensation Program was created under similarly turbulent and perilous circumstances.[5] Lawsuits against vaccine manufacturers had soared during the litigious 1970s and '80s. In particular, lawsuits related to the (ultimately discredited) theory of vaccine-induced autism terrified manufacturers. Because the profit margin on vaccines wasn't very large to begin with, many companies undertook a brass tacks analysis and decided it simply wasn't worth the effort. One by one, manufacturers ceased producing vaccines. There was the very real threat of complete loss of childhood vaccines.

Like the image of pregnant women being turned away, the image of thousands of children newly paralyzed by polio or stricken by the illnesses of generations past did not play well in the public arena. Congress was forced to act and created the National Vaccine Injury Compensation Program. This allowed families to get compensated for injuries related to childhood vaccines, though only for those side effects that had scientific documentation. Shielded from bankrupting lawsuits, manufacturers could resume producing vaccines. (A number of companies, however, did not return to the field. The legacy remains today, with many vaccines produced by only one or two companies, leaving the public susceptible to both shortages and price inflation.)

Like the Danish system, these American programs are no-fault systems—the patient does not have to prove negligence. The case is adjudicated by an administrative panel and if the injury is felt to be related to the birth or the vaccine, there is a payout. In general, these programs have been considered reasonably successful in that costs were controlled, injured patents received compensation, and the respective insurance and vaccine emergencies were stabilized. While the Danish system is funded by the public, the vaccine fund is financed by a small fee on all vaccines (which, it could be argued, is the public). The birth-injury funds come from fees on doctors, hospitals, and insurers.

So, could this model work on a more comprehensive scale? Could the United States take the Nordic plunge and move from the litigation system to a no-fault compensation system? Michelle Mello is a legal scholar at Stanford University who spent years investigating this possibility, an idea that has come to be called "health courts."[6] Like worker's compensation, this injury compensation system—despite its moniker—would exist outside the courts, using specially trained administrators. Rather than having to prove negligence, patients would only have to show that an injury would have been avoidable (preventable) if best practices had been in place. Using guidelines for common medical errors and injuries, a significant portion of cases could be adjudicated quickly and without the need for lawyers.

When I asked Mello what the biggest barrier to health courts is, she laughed and said, "Trial lawyers." Removing these cases from the regular courts and reducing the need for legal representation would remove a significant slice of income for lawyers.

In 2010, when a consideration for health courts was floated as part of the Affordable Care Act, a spokesperson for the American Association for Justice stated: "Health courts would involve the creation of an outrageously expensive new bureaucracy to handle the very few medical negligence claims that exist today. . . . It will do nothing to eliminate the 98,000 people who die every year from preventable medical errors."[7] You will not be surprised to learn that the unassumingly named American Association for Justice used to be known as the Association of Trial Lawyers of America.

A major advantage of health courts is that they would introduce a measure of consistency: comparable injuries would be treated in a standardized way. There would be accepted standards both for which kinds of injuries should be compensated and how much should be paid out. This stands in contrast to settlements negotiated by lawyers (or decided by juries), which vary wildly.

Moreover, the health courts, in Mello's opinion, "would be tied to patient safety as well as cost savings." Because they have the potential to bring a broader and more representative sample of patient injury to light—not just the catastrophic cases that malpractice suits highlight—the healthcare system would receive more accurate signals about what needs to be improved.

But the strongest selling point of health courts—and the driving force behind the Danish switch—is simple fairness. It would allow many more patients to get compensation and get it faster than in our current litigation-based system, even if the payouts are lower.

However, the perception that a jury of one's peers protects the average person is tightly woven into the American fabric, even if few people are actually able to get their day in court. Mello observes, "Congress always says, 'We need juries to protect the little guy,' but 80% of the time the little guy loses jury trials." Of course, this romantic attachment to juries might just be a fig leaf for underlying financial interests. After all, Mello notes, "many lawmakers used to be trial lawyers."

Given that the malpractice system remains the primary construct for addressing patient harm, at least in the US, one question is whether it might be reformed in such a way that its objectives could be better aligned with the wider goal of patient safety. Michelle Mello and her colleague Allen Kachalia have proposed a number of intriguing reforms that might help the malpractice system improve overall safety, while still addressing the needs of the individual patient who brought the suit.[8] One example is holding the *institution* liable in addition to (or instead of) the individual clinician. This acknowledges the fact—as Lucian Leape forcefully pointed out—that there's almost always a systems problem that enabled a human to make an error. Besides forcing institutions to keep more skin in the game financially, settlements would also include mandates to fix the systems issues (in addition to whatever payout the individual patient might receive).

Another suggestion involves the malpractice insurance that doctors and hospitals must hold. As we saw in Florida and Virginia, the spiraling cost of insurance—which is steeper for high-risk specialties—can make health-care less safe, especially if all the doctors quit practice! But perhaps insurance rates could be subsidized by the government for institutions that meet certain patient-safety goals. This could channel the threat of malpractice into more productive avenues that have the potential to improve the entire system.

Then there is the larger question about whether the legal system—either through malpractice suits or with administrative health courts—is the best place to resolve medical errors. Might it be possible to handle errors entirely within the medical system itself? Rather than have patients and doctors duke it out as opposing teams, could there be a way for patients to obtain the information they need, receive a payout if appropriate, and have doctors be able to acknowledge and apologize for the error without everyone having to be dragged through the coals?

Over the course of several years, Michelle Mello's research led her to something called Communication and Resolution Programs (CRPs), which I'll discuss toward the end of the case I present in the next chapter. Like Mello, this family eventually found its way to CRPs, but via a more convoluted—and far more painful—route.

# CHAPTER THIRTEEN

# LOOKING FOR ANSWERS

In this marriage (at least for the past two decades of their forty-six years together), there was a clear division of labor: Nancy was in charge of the yardwork and flowers and Glenn was the fruits-and-vegetables man. Glenn planted apple, peach, and pear trees along with raspberries, blueberries, blackberries, and grape vines, plus enough tomatoes, green beans, and squash to feed the entire neighborhood and then some. As a science teacher, Glenn never lost his sense of wonderment about the environment. If there was an oddball pack of seeds that promised gourds with shapes resembling modern art installations, he'd be first to try them. Even when he became a principal, his first task upon returning home at the end of the day would be to walk the garden and see what needed to be pruned, harvested, or otherwise coaxed to life from the temperamental Kansas soil.

Glenn was also an enthusiastic woodworker, scrounging scrap wood or convincing construction workers to donate their leftovers so he could create toy cars and planes. Whenever the fruits of his woodworking and the fruits of his garden piled up, he and Nancy would haul the lot to a local farmers' market to sell or even give away. "He just loved doing things for kids and working with wood," Nancy, an elementary school teacher, told me. When their daughter Melissa was four, she requested a workbench for Christmas. Glenn fashioned a tiny one, complete with working tools to fit a four-year-old's hands. (When Melissa asked for power tools the following Christmas, Glenn demurred. Those didn't show up as a Christmas gift until Melissa was in college.)

Two minutes from Glenn and Nancy's home was a sparkling, spring-fed lake, hemmed in by a 500-foot-long earthen dam that protected the downhill homes from being inundated with water. In rural Kansas, dam maintenance is left to the local communities, which must abide by state regulations and pass regular inspections, and Glenn was part of the homeowners' association committee that cared for their dam. One of the challenges of an earthen dam is keeping out tree roots and local critters, both of whose burrowing will weaken the dam. To achieve this, the state encourages a "controlled burn" every year to clear away brush, trees, and by extension any animals who might view such fauna as prime real estate for family living.

On a late afternoon at the end of March, Glenn and his neighbors were preparing for the annual burn. Most had done this together for several years, though the prior year there'd been a moratorium on fires because of drought conditions. That moratorium meant that the underbrush was twice as thick this year. And it was all made worse by an outbreak of the invasive weed Johnsongrass, whose tenacious stalks can shoot up to seven feet tall and whose roots form an insidious underground network of botanical contagion.

An overflow pipe in the dam prevented the lake from spilling over, especially during heavy rains. The outflow from this pipe created a shallow stream on the dry side of the dam, toward the west end of the 500-foot embankment. It was near this stream that Glenn and his partner were tackling overgrown brush with gas-powered weed cutters. It was essential to clear the brush around the pipe so the fire wouldn't edge too close and melt the liner of the pipe.

For a man in his late sixties, Glenn was in excellent shape. His gardening passion kept him outdoors and working his entire life, and he had no trouble mustering up the necessary elbow grease needed to wrestle the brush and manage the fire. The plan was for one team to start the main fire on the east end of the dam; this fire would move west and up over the dam into the lake. A backfire would then be started on the west end of the dam, closer to where the outflow pipe protruded. This fire would move east and up toward the top of the dam.

What happened next wasn't exactly clear—Glenn later told Nancy that he thought the backfire had been started too soon—but the area near the stream ignited and flames shot up around the two men. Glenn's partner was able to escape to the road that paralleled the dam. Realizing he couldn't evade the fire, Glenn threw himself down into the tiny stream from the overflow pipe, immersing himself as best he could in the shallow water.

This strategy worked. When Glenn climbed out of the stream he knew that the left side of his face had been burned but that he was essentially okay. Glenn's biggest frustration from all of this was that his glasses were missing by the time he pulled himself out of the stream. He dug around in the mud for a few minutes, but it was hopeless. He gave up and walked over to the road, climbing into the bed of his truck. One of the other men drove him the two minutes to home.

Glenn was a sooty, drippy mess at the door, and Nancy remembered that he looked like he'd just emerged from one of those 1950s swamp movies. Glenn's first question was, "Do I have any eyebrows left?" She assured him that he did, but looking at his singed face, she suggested they ought to go to the hospital, just to get him checked out.

They agreed that Glenn should at least rinse off a few layers of soot first. Nancy helped peel off his muddy knee-high boots. Glenn put them in the garage so they wouldn't mess up the house and then headed to the shower. When Glenn took off his soggy blackened clothes in the bathroom, he saw that his back was burned and blistered too. So post-shower, in his robe and slippers, he climbed into the passenger seat of their car and Nancy drove him to the local hospital ten minutes away. There were only two stop signs on the route, but Glenn told her not to stop.

"Stay here," she said to Glenn when they arrived, and she hurried to the ER entrance to request a wheelchair. There wasn't one readily available, but a young man in the waiting area offered to help. Before they could even get out the door, though, there was Glenn padding through the parking lot in his bedroom slippers and dark-blue robe with the gray trim. It was nearly 6:30 p.m., but the sky still wielded its afternoon brightness, thanks to daylight savings time.

The ER nurse quickly triaged Glenn. "He'll most likely have to go to the burn center," she said. *Burn center* sounded serious, Nancy remembered thinking. He'd probably have to be airlifted out of state to Denver or Dallas.

But when the ER doctor examined Glenn, he was more reassuring. "The burns aren't bad enough to go to the burn center," he told Nancy. "But we will admit him to our ICU." Nancy, who was still dazed from all of the events, found tentative relief: things weren't so bad. She wondered, though, whether Glenn would have any scarring on his face from the burns. But what a plus that he would be so close to home, not hours away in another state.

The local hospital was new, or at least the building was brand-new. The defining medical challenge for rural hospitals has always been attracting— and retaining—enough doctors. Far-flung sleepy towns can be a hard sell to doctors, who tend to congregate in the urban centers where they'd trained. So new medical facilities with high-end services such as ICUs were springing up, betting that these could entice doctors from the big cities.

This emergency room, like many ERs in small towns, was covered by a rotation of the hospital's doctors. This model was, in fact, standard practice throughout the entire country before emergency medicine became a recognized medical specialty in 1979. Most larger hospitals are now staffed with full-time emergency medicine doctors, but rural hospitals have to make do with the old system.

Similarly, the ICU was not staffed by 24-hour critical-care specialists; it also relied on a rotation of doctors. In fact, the ICU had to be opened up to admit Glenn. It was already late in the evening when he arrived from the ER. While hooking up Glenn's IVs, the ICU nurse turned to Nancy and said, "I'm going to try and get him transferred to the burn center." That's when Nancy learned that the burn center was only one hour away in Wichita, not out of state as she'd thought.

---

When burn victims come to medical attention they are assessed in two ways—*severity* of burns and *extent* of burns. Severity is determined by the depth of the burn in relation to the skin and underlying tissue: superficial (first-degree), partial-thickness (second-degree), or full-thickness (third-degree). Extent is determined by percentage of the body affected. The rule of nines is a quick way to roughly estimate the percentage of surface area burned—the arms and head are each 9% and the legs, chest, and back are each 18%.

The deeper the burns and the greater the percentage of the body involved, the more serious the situation is. Glenn had burns on parts of his face, chest, back, and abdomen. The initial estimate in the ER was that 30% of his body-surface area was affected and that these were second-degree (partial-thickness) burns.

The principles of burn treatment rest on four major pillars. The first is securing an airway, since smoke inhalation is highly toxic to the lungs. Additionally, the vast fluid shifts that take place after burns can cause airways to swell and close off. Severely burned patients are therefore usually intubated immediately and placed on a ventilator.

The second pillar is hydration, since skin is the major barrier that keeps our fluids inside of us. Patients with second- and third-degree burns always need fluids in order to maintain enough volume coursing through the blood vessels to keep the kidneys and brain functioning. But fluid management needs to be done with extreme care, since the inflammatory cascade set off by burn injuries makes the vessels "leaky." Much of the IV fluid can end up pooling in the tissues if not carefully titrated. This is not only useless—in terms of getting blood volume to critical organs—it's also harmful. Edematous, boggy tissue at the site of the burns impedes healing. It can also cause further skin breakdown, infection, and impaired circulation.

For these reasons, there are precise calculations for fluid administration that take into account body size and burn size, but then also shift over time to match the time course of the body's inflammatory reaction. But even these exacting formulas are only estimates, as the hydration needs to be titrated to the realities of each patient. The fluids have to be adjusted individually for each patient to ensure that the flow is high enough for that patient's organs to work (e.g., to get steady urine output from the kidneys) but also low enough to prevent excess fluid buildup near the burns and in the lungs. The complexity of fluid management is one of the primary reasons that burn centers were developed.

The third pillar of burn treatment is prevention of infection, since loss of skin is a floodgate invitation to all of our bacterial neighbors. Burns require exquisite care to avoid contamination and that care can never slip up, not even for a second. (You will likely never meet a more fanatically obsessive person than a burn-unit nurse in charge of dressing changes.)

The fourth pillar is pain management. Burns rank among the most painful of human experiences. Deeper burns may not be painful themselves because the nerves have been charred, but the dressing changes are notoriously excruciating. Some burn patients will tell you that they've considered suicide as a very reasonable option during their treatments, just to escape the pain.

------

That night in the ICU was a rocky one for Glenn. He was endlessly thirsty and kept asking Nancy for ice chips. But his blood pressure was falling, and his kidneys were struggling. He was on a host of medications, including antibiotics, steroids, opiates for pain, and anti-nausea meds. By the time pressors (the sledgehammer medications to boost blood pressure) were started, he'd stopped talking. When their local pastor came by for a visit just past midnight, he was no longer responsive.

In the morning, Glenn was transferred to the burn center in Wichita; Nancy arrived shortly thereafter. The doctor at the burn center was not one to mince words. He told Nancy three things right off the bat: "Glenn should have been transferred to the burn center immediately." "He didn't get enough fluids." "I expect him to die before the day is out."

For Nancy, this was almost impossible to comprehend. The evening before, Glenn had walked himself to the ER in his bathrobe. He'd been asking for ice chips in the ICU. Now he was expected to die before the day was out?

The doctor turned out to be correct on his first statement, largely correct on the second, and wrong on the third—though, sadly, not wrong enough.

Glenn never regained consciousness, although his robust body powered him through ten more days of intensive, exhausting treatment. Dialysis revived his kidneys but could not save him. The damage to his brain and other organs was too extensive. On April 11, a doctor Nancy had never met before made the recommendation to remove life support. After consultation with her two adult children and with the medical team, Nancy made the hardest decision of her life and signed the papers to remove life support. Her husband of forty-six years died within minutes.

What drew me to Glenn's story wasn't the intricacies of burn management so much as the intricacies of *error* management: what happens *after* an error has occurred. In particular, how do patients and families get information in order to understand what happened?

The errors that took place during Glenn's initial care could probably be explained in less than ten minutes. But it took nearly four years for his family to extract this information from the hospital. The excruciating, slogging-through-tar journey that Glenn's family experienced is a regrettably common one. Everyone has stories about battling bureaucracies at the DMV or in government agencies but nothing quite compares to attempting to penetrate the healthcare bureaucracy in the setting of a major medical error.

It's entirely possible that Glenn might have died even if he had been transferred to the burn unit immediately. Indeed, this is one of the most challenging aspects of evaluating a medical error—establishing causality. And it's one of the biggest critiques of the studies that have tried to determine the number of deaths from medical error. Many patients experience errors and many of these patients die, but that is a long way from saying that the patients died *because* of the medical error. Errors naturally congregate around very sick patients because their medical care has exponentially more moving parts and thus more opportunity—statistically speaking—to experience errors. With complicated cases it can be impossible to tease out whether the error caused the death or whether the severe underlying illness caused the death, with the error just riding alongside.

There's no doubt that Glenn should have been transferred to a burn center immediately. And there were other errors in Glenn's care that came to light later. Whether these errors actually caused his death, though, is not possible to say with certainty. What *is* possible to say with certainty, however, is that a beloved man was ripped from his family, leaving a gaping, ragged wound that no protocol or algorithm or lawsuit could ever heal.

At the time of the accident, Glenn and Nancy's daughter Melissa was out on the West Coast pursuing a PhD in biomedical informatics. Melissa had arrived at this field after a peripatetic student career that wound its way from cell biology to design and then eventually to biomedical informatics. She was intrigued by how one could use the principles of design to structure biomedical information in a way that's easier for people to understand.

It turns out that having a PhD in the science of information in biomedicine doesn't make it any easier to get information from the medical system. After Glenn's death, Melissa was just as stunned and confused as her mother. Based on that first-day comment from the doctor at the burn center, Melissa and Nancy wanted to know why their local hospital hadn't transferred Glenn immediately. You didn't need a PhD (or an MD, for that matter) to look up the transfer criteria on the American Burn Society website. It took Melissa about ten seconds to find the guidelines and it all seemed rather straightforward—anyone with second-degree burns on 30% of their body should be transferred.

Melissa and Nancy weren't necessarily interested in suing the hospital over this. They just wanted to know why Glenn's doctors had decided not to transfer him. They both recognized that medicine is a complex field and that human beings don't always fit the textbook. Maybe there were complicated shades of gray in Glenn's case? Maybe someone worried about the risks of transferring an unstable patient in the middle of the night? Maybe there was a logistical reason the transfer couldn't be accommodated? They wanted to understand what had happened and why. And they wanted to be sure that the next burn victim who arrived in the ER would get the appropriate treatment. To them, this seemed like basic information that any hospital where a tragic outcome had occurred should be willing to provide for the family. Melissa and Nancy soon learned that a 500-foot earthen dam that holds back an entire lake was a collection of mere toothpicks compared to the wall that holds back a hospital's information when there is fear of a lawsuit.

Graduate students reside at the low end of the heap in most aspects of departmental hierarchy but nowhere more so than in real estate. Offices for graduate students were out of the question in Melissa's department. So, too, it seemed, were cubicles. But she was able to score a desk in a hallway, surrounded by faculty offices and the daily departmental traffic.

Melissa had returned to school after her father's funeral but it was impossible to step right back into her studies. There was still the disorienting amalgam of emotions, the surrealness of a sudden absence of someone who had always been so present. And then there were the myriad questions still hanging like daggers in the air: Why hadn't Glenn been transferred to the burn center immediately? Did the local hospital realize its error? Was it doing anything about it?

From her studies, Melissa knew that any serious medical error should trigger an internal investigation. She wondered if the hospital considered what had happened to her father to be serious? Had they made changes to their procedures so that this wouldn't happen to the next patient? Did they even care?

Melissa spent hours parked at her hallway desk, thinking not about her PhD work but rather about how to get answers about her father. How could her family get the information they needed in order to grapple with the enormity of losing Glenn? How could they begin to knit their lives back together without fully understanding his death?

Melissa realized that the location of her humble hallway desk was actually a resource. Not everyone who suffers in the wake of a medical error has the ironic fortune to be situated in medical school, in a department devoted to medical information, no less. Melissa sought out her professors and posed her question: what does a family do when they want to find out information from a hospital after a medical error? The professors referred her to Tom Gallagher, a religion major who segued into bioethics and became an internist at the University of Washington with an expertise in medical error. Gallagher advised Melissa to request a meeting with the hospital CEO. But he warned her that, given the pervasive fear of lawsuits, the hospital would likely be cagey in its responses.

That warning turned out to be simultaneously an understatement and prophetic. Approximately six weeks after Glenn's death, Melissa and Nancy found themselves sitting in the office of the hospital CEO. They had invited a local pastor to the meeting, hoping that would lessen the tension. It didn't.

For Melissa and Nancy, this meeting was about Glenn. But you wouldn't have known that if you'd transcribed the words of the CEO. Other than an obligatory "I'm sorry for your loss," Glenn never came up at all. The CEO didn't even seem to acknowledge that Glenn had been a patient in his hospital. It was as though Glenn—arguably the raison d'être of this meeting—didn't exist at all.

Nancy described to the CEO her experience of watching her husband suffer, of watching the nurses frantically trying to get Glenn transferred. The body language of the CEO may not have been deliberate, but it remains imprinted on Melissa's memory: "He leaned back in his chair and waved his hand like he was shooing away a fly."

The CEO informed Nancy and Melissa that the hospital was prevented—by law—from discussing the details of Glenn's care with them. According to him, medical records and details could not be shared. Both Nancy and Melissa recalled being almost too stunned to reply. *Really?* The hospital couldn't tell the family of the patient who died anything at all?

After the meeting, Nancy and Melissa mulled over this and wondered if perhaps the hospital was still in a state of confusion over the events, or maybe it was still in the middle of its own internal review. That could conceivably explain its reticence to reveal details. But they felt that their request was reasonable enough—they just wanted to understand what had happened to their husband and father. So they wrote a letter to the CEO, outlining their concerns. They inquired whether the case had been reported to the state and wanted to know what corrective measures were being taken.

The reply from the CEO reiterated that the law "specifically precludes us from disclosing information with outside parties." *Outside parties?* The immediate family was considered an outside party? "Many of the issues raised in your letter," the CEO wrote, "cannot be disclosed or discussed."

Nancy and Melissa found this perplexing and decided to take a look at the law. The wording of the statute was dense but the gist seemed to be that internal reviews of adverse events could not be subpoenaed in a court of law. Internal reviews could be used only for disciplinary hearings by the appropriate licensing board. Presumably, this law was passed so that fear of litigation would not discourage hospitals from examining their medical errors. However, there was nothing that Nancy or Melissa could see in the law that prohibited talking with *families.*

It was October before Nancy secured another meeting with the CEO. This time there was a hospital lawyer present along with a member of the hospital's board. But she got the same response—state law prevented them from releasing information. The upshot of what they said was: "If you want us to talk to you, you have to get the law changed." Oddly enough, they even offered to assist.

Over the next few months, Nancy tried to stay in touch with the CEO, and even met with him again, but obtained almost no information. He did say that he agreed that hospitals should be able to talk to patients and families about medical errors, that it was unfortunate that the law prevented this. The one thing Nancy did learn was that the nursing staff had continued to advocate for Glenn to be transferred to the burn center over the course of his night in the ICU. At least that was something, but no other details were forthcoming. Melissa was convinced that the CEO's offer to help write a new law was just a stalling tactic. What an ingenious way to get pestering families off your back—send them off to change the state legal code. That'll keep 'em occupied for a few years.

But Melissa and her mother Nancy were not deterred. If changing the state law was what was required to breech the wall of silence around the hospital, so be it. Toward the end of that year, they began drafting their first bill to require hospitals to disclose serious medical errors to patients and families. They didn't want a law that simply gave hospitals *permission* to talk to patients and families, they wanted hospitals to be *required* to disclose information about medical errors. The hospital CEO arranged a meeting with their state representative, who agreed to introduce the bill.

Meanwhile, since no further information was forthcoming from the hospital, Nancy filed formal complaints with the Kansas Board of Healing Arts (the state licensing organization) as well as the Kansas Foundation for Medical Care (a quality-improvement program authorized by Medicare).

After three months, the Kansas Foundation replied with a letter stating, "We determined that some of the care your husband received did not meet professionally recognized standards of care." But that admission turned out to be the full extent of the information that would be shared with Melissa and Nancy. No details. No conclusions. And no action.

The Kansas Board of Healing Arts undertook an investigation. This was the most promising lead, a true medical investigation into Glenn's medical care. Finally there would be some answers, Melissa and Nancy thought. However, they were informed that the results of the investigation would be made available only if disciplinary action was ultimately recommended. Otherwise the results would be sealed.

The investigation took a full year. Melissa and Nancy held cautious hope that this would be a detailed analysis and that they would finally learn what transpired during Glenn's one night at the hospital. After a year of waiting, the investigation was concluded, and Nancy received the following reply: "Based upon the Disciplinary Panel's review of the evidence in the investigation and a thorough legal analysis, public disciplinary action was not authorized." And that was it. Case closed.

All sorts of people seemed to be able to evaluate the details of Glenn's medical care—the doctors, the hospital administrators, the state licensing board, Medicare's quality-improvement foundation. The only "party" not privy to Glenn's information, it seemed, was Glenn's family.

When Melissa was a first-year PhD student, she'd sat through the requisite lectures about medical error. She recalled that it was an uncomfortable topic. "It wasn't something that I wanted to think about," she said. Looking back at it later, though, it dawned on her that medical error as an educational topic was presented only from the perspective of the healthcare system—the doctors, nurses, and hospitals. Never from the patients' perspective. All the teaching, research, and policy work about medical errors came from the side that *committed* the errors, not the side that experienced the errors.

In Melissa's program—as in most others—errors were taught as problems to be solved, problems to be prevented. Important, yes, but the errors weren't ever presented as the harm that patients and their families experienced. They weren't presented as the death and devastation that destroyed peoples' lives. There wasn't a hint of the anguish that Melissa and Nancy were experiencing now.

When Melissa thinks about herself during those introductory lectures, she sees an almost laughable innocence in how her younger self could just brush away those annoying required topics. "Who would want to think about medical error? It never occurred to me that I could be on the receiving end," she told me.

But now she and her mother were faced with a difficult decision. Kansas law states that medical malpractice lawsuits must be filed no more than two years from the date of injury. If they wanted to file a lawsuit they would have to do so before the statute of limitations ran out. They could hardly envision a less desirable project to take on in their lives. But what else could they do? It had been almost two years since Glenn died and they still had no idea what transpired on that first night in the hospital.

Filing a malpractice lawsuit requires energy and fight—things that are in notable short supply when you are grieving the death of someone you love. But there seemed to be no other way. "And we were fortunate," Melissa said, fully aware of the irony of that word, "because we could show that there was harm done, that there was negligence on the part of the hospital, and that the negligence caused the harm." And because the outcome was horrific enough—death—their case earned the malpractice prize of being "financially viable." Melissa and Nancy knew that the overwhelming majority of people who'd experienced harm were not able to pursue litigation because their cases didn't meet all the criteria.

What they did not know, however, was how traumatic and exhausting the lawsuit process would be. Once Nancy decided to proceed with a lawsuit—just before the statute of limitations expired—it was ten long months before pretrial depositions could even begin. And once the depositions started, it took another ten months to complete them, during which time Nancy and Melissa each had to testify, along with Melissa's brother, two family friends,

plus four nurses, three doctors, one physician assistant, one hospital administrator, and five expert witnesses.

"Grueling" would be an understatement. Nancy's questioning lasted a
full eight-hour day. So did Melissa's. Some of the questions asked of them
seemed pointless and repetitive. When Melissa tabulated how many pages
of testimony were generated by the depositions, she noticed that her and her
mother's testimonies were more than twice as long as the doctors' and nurses'.
They equaled and even exceeded the testimonies of the expert witnesses. As a
graduate student and an elementary school teacher, neither of whom participated in Glenn's medical care or had the slightest expertise to offer, it seemed
curious that the hospitals' lawyers had such a volume of questions for them.
In Melissa's opinion it was a strategic assault, a way to wear down the family,
maybe even punish them for pursuing a lawsuit, not to mention a convenient
way to rack up billable hours.

It took almost two further years—on top of the two years Melissa and
Nancy had already spent trying to get information—but the lawsuit was finally negotiated to an ending without having to go to court. Melissa and
Nancy aren't allowed to discuss the terms of what the parties agreed upon, but
over the course of the process, they finally learned what happened to Glenn
during his overnight stay at their local hospital.

They'd already known about the first error that had taken place—the failure to transfer Glenn immediately to a burn center. The second major error
they learned about was the fluid management. The burn center doctor had
been partly correct about Glenn not getting enough fluids, but the mismanagement turned out to be far more complicated than that. Glenn received the
wrong type of fluid as well as the wrong amounts of fluid at the wrong times.

For burn victims, the recommended type of fluid is lactated Ringer's solution, but Glenn received dextrose saline. Glenn's blood sugar subsequently
skyrocketed, and he required insulin treatment at the burn center to bring it
down. The larger error in Glenn's fluid management, though, was that the rate
was not carefully titrated during that first night. Although there is a tempta-
tion to give as much fluid as possible, as fast as possible, for these severely dehydrated patients, burn protocols are very careful in the initial hours, because
the vessels are at their leakiest due to the body's seismic inflammatory reaction
to the burn.

When Glenn first arrived in the ER, he was given boluses of the dextrose saline. This overly aggressive amount of IV fluid swamped his leaky vessels, inundating and damaging the surrounding tissues. One expert witness
concluded that some of Glenn's second-degree (partial-thickness) burns were
converted to third-degree (full-thickness) by the excessive fluid and swelling

in the tissues. (The standard formula does recommend higher rates of fluid administration in the first eight hours but does not recommend boluses of fluid.)

The burn-center doctor's assessment that Glenn didn't get enough fluids was ultimately correct, though, in the physiologic sense—Glenn's blood vessels didn't have enough fluid inside of them. So even though Glenn was receiving liters and liters of fluid, very little stayed inside his vessels, and he ultimately went into hypovolemic shock: there was not enough volume of fluid inside the vessels to reach the critical organs. (This highlights that the most important tenet of fluid management is not adherence to the standard-of-care formula—no matter how sophisticated that formula is—but careful titration of fluids to the functioning of the organs in each individual patient, especially to urine output and neurologic functioning.)

Compounding the problem, however, was that in response to this hypovolemic shock that Glenn was experiencing in the ICU, the medical team chose to administer pressors. Pressors (sometimes called vasopressors) squeeze the vessels tighter in order to jack up the blood pressure. Using these drugs make sense for some instances of low blood pressure, but if there's not enough fluid inside the vessels, giving pressors is like gunning a car that's out of gas.

Not only are pressors ineffective in these situations, but they are also potentially damaging. By squeezing the vessels tight, they can render it impossible for what little fluid there is to move forward. Sensitive organs such as the kidneys are often the first to go in scenarios like this, which is precisely what happened to Glenn that night. This led to another medical error.

When Glenn's urine output began to decrease, the ER doctor responded by ordering a dose of a diuretic. A diuretic can indeed push a kidney to make more urine, but it can only do this with a functioning kidney. If the kidney is faltering because it's lacking oxygen from decreased blood flow, you can throw on a Niagara Falls' worth of diuretics, but little will happen. The same analogy of gunning a car without gas holds here.

There were a number of other errors in Glenn's care that night. Glenn probably should have been intubated immediately on arrival, given the extent of his burns and the high probability of an unstable course ahead. Glenn was also given a dose of steroids. While steroids are occasionally used in treating septic shock related to an infection—though guardedly, because they are a double-edged sword—they have no role in hypovolemic shock.

For pain, Glenn was prescribed patient-controlled anesthesia—an IV setup that allows the patient to press a button to deliver pain medication when needed. This arrangement is excellent for a patient with a broken leg. But within hours of arrival to the ICU, Glenn was hardly conscious and was in no condition to be adjusting his own pain meds. While this would not be a life-threatening error, it does suggest that no one was examining the patient carefully.

Beyond the above errors in treatment, there were also errors of judgment. The nurses caring for Glenn in the ICU contacted the on-call doctor that night to try to get Glenn transferred to the burn center, but the doctor decided against the transfer and instead gave medication orders by phone. He chose not to drive the five minutes to the hospital to evaluate the patient in person. While there are certainly many medical situations that can be handled safely by phone, any patient sick enough to warrant admission to an intensive care unit is sick enough to warrant a full evaluation. Especially if there are no other physicians on site—no team of medical residents who can be the eyes and ears on the ground, no cardiology fellows, pulmonary fellows, or renal fellows to handle the complications. Thus, Glenn's first night of ICU care was based on the initial impression of the ER doctor (who was not an emergency-medicine specialist) and then phone conversations with a doctor from home who did not personally evaluate the patient.

The litany of medical errors that unfolded during the deposition testimonies of the doctors and nurses was shocking to Nancy and Melissa. No wonder the hospital resisted revealing the details of Glenn's care. The conclusion from the Kansas Foundation for Medical Care that "some of the care your husband received did not meet professionally recognized standards of care" was an understatement of Kansas-prairie proportions.

But the real horror for Glenn's family was learning the details of the communications among the staff during that night. The first ER nurse had told Nancy that Glenn would likely be transferred to the burn center, but then the ER doctor said it wasn't necessary. What Nancy and Melissa later learned was that someone in the ER had pulled out the guidelines for transfer to a burn center from the hospital's collection of policy manuals. The house supervisor (the head nurse for the hospital that night) had photocopied the page, emphasized the transfer criteria with a highlighter pen, and then handed it to the ER doctor. The doctor still declined to transfer Glenn.

That first ER nurse didn't stand up to the doctor, even though she disagreed with his clinical assessment. In her testimony, she stated that "she would never go against what a doctor said."

The house supervisor, though, continued to lobby for transfer. He phoned the on-call administrator. Typically, this role is rotated among the different members of the senior leadership team of the hospital, some of whom have clinical backgrounds and some of whom come from the management world. On this night the on-call administrator happened to be the Director of Nursing. Nancy and Melissa assumed that the Director of Nursing would have backed up the house supervisor (the head nurse) in his efforts to convince the ER doctor to transfer Glenn to the burn center. Instead, she declined to call the doctor, saying that it wouldn't do any good. (The house supervisor went to the CEO first thing Monday morning to report what had transpired.)

The overnight ICU nurse testified that she did not feel qualified to handle a patient with an illness of Glenn's severity, and that she was essentially alone on that first night, since the on-call doctor had declined to come to the hospital. When the day-shift ICU nurse showed up the next morning, she was apparently shocked at what was going on. Her first words were something along the lines of, "Why hasn't this patient been transferred to the burn center?" She immediately called the PA (physician assistant) covering the ICU for the day, who had Glenn intubated on the spot. The PA called Glenn's primary care doctor, who agreed to transfer Glenn to the burn center, and the transfer took place later that morning.

Glenn died eleven days later.

---

"I trusted the doctors," Nancy told me. "I trusted the hospital." But the weeks and months of testimony were as eye-opening as they were gut-wrenching. To learn that some of the staff were fighting desperately to get Glenn the care he needed, only to be overruled by others, was simply crushing. Nancy recalled an article she'd seen in the local newspaper when the new hospital building had opened. It said one of the benefits of the new facility was that they could keep more patients there, rather than transferring them to larger hospitals.

Nancy isn't an intrinsically conspiracy-minded person. But she couldn't help wondering whether money played a role. Were the staff discouraged from transferring patients? Were there quiet pressures to keep patients in-house? Though maybe it wasn't about money at all. Maybe some of the people caring for Glenn were not competent or, at the very least, were in over their heads. Alternatively, the problems could have stemmed from the hospital's culture. Perhaps this hospital had a culture in which it was not acceptable to admit ignorance or ask for help. Maybe the hierarchies were so ingrained that there was simply no acceptable way for a decision to be questioned, even by competent and caring staff.

Melissa and Nancy both understood that Glenn's injuries had been severe and that he might have died even if he'd been transferred to the burn center immediately. They even understood that mistakes sometimes happen, even tragic ones. What they couldn't understand—or accept—was that they'd had to fight for nearly four years to fully learn what happened. Those years should have been theirs to dwell on their grief, their love, and the long, brambled road toward healing. Those years should have been theirs to decide how to mourn. Instead they'd had to fight.

"Not once during the whole process," Melissa told me, "did anyone sit down with us and lay out what happened. We had to piece it together ourselves from the depositions." Among other things, the struggle for information wrenched a hole in Melissa's PhD program. It was just too much to balance classes with what became a second job—making phone calls, writing letters, keeping up with the depositions, and, of course, tending to the excruciating sadness in the family.

Melissa had begun reading up on medical error shortly after her father's death. One of the cultural shifts over the past twenty years was the recognition that doctors need to openly acknowledge error and apologize directly to patients. Some states had even passed laws that offered legal protections to doctors, so that honest apologies couldn't be used against them. To Melissa, this felt demeaning to the patients. It was as though all the concern was directed toward making things easier for doctors. They had the option of apologizing but no requirement to disclose information. Everything was from the doctor's perspective. What about the patient and family?

Melissa and Nancy realized they were going to have to roll up their sleeves on this, even more than they were already doing for Glenn's individual case. They had begun drafting a legislative bill in the months after Glenn's death—based on work by Tom Gallagher and his colleagues[1]—and they were determined to make it law. There had to be a legal way for patients and families to obtain information from hospitals.

Advocating for their legislation was a laborious process. Melissa arranged phone calls with representatives from medical and legal associations. Nancy schlepped back and forth to Topeka to meet with state representatives and government officials, explaining the situation over and over again. Patient-advocacy groups didn't exist in Kansas, so lawmakers had always taken their cues from medical organizations. Staking a claim from the patient perspective was an uphill battle.

State politics is always a rough-and-tumble, unforgiving setting for reasoned analysis, but Kansas was in the throes of a particularly high-voltage battle over the state budget. An unpopular governor had slashed funding for schools and public services to make up for a gaping hole in the state budget, and nearly everyone everywhere was enraged about something. It took two full years, but their bill finally secured a hearing in the Kansas House Judiciary Committee.

Three major medical organizations were also present to push a separate bill focused on protecting doctors' apologies from being used against them.

Nancy and Melissa's bill included this protection, but it also contained a mandate to disclose serious medical errors to patients. Nancy and Melissa had hoped that they could collaborate with the medical organizations to develop a bill that addressed everyone's concerns. When all three medical groups rose to testify *against* their bill, however, they realized that this was wishful thinking.

In the end, neither bill made it out of committee. "Legislators told me to keep trying," Nancy said. "They said these things take years." Undaunted, Nancy and Melissa drafted a second bill. This one focused solely on disclosure of medical errors to patients and families. It took another two years for their second bill to gain a hearing, this time by the Senate Judiciary Committee. But again, the medical organizations opposed it, submitting written testimonies against it. Melissa told me, "I think they were saying, 'We have our own way of doing things. We don't want anyone telling us what to do.'"

Neither of their bills made it to the House or Senate floor for a vote. But along their legislative journey, Nancy and Melissa found that nearly everyone they spoke with—either while lobbying or just in their everyday lives— had their own brush with medical error. Whether it concerned themselves, a relative, or a friend, there was always a medical horror story readily at hand. Medical error and patient harm seemed nearly universal.

Since the legislative front wasn't succeeding, it was time to try something else. Nancy flew out to Seattle to visit Melissa and asked to meet Tom Gallagher. I had interviewed Gallagher for this book long before I'd come across Glenn's story and Melissa and Nancy's journey. So it was somewhat unexpected to have these two strands of research come together.

---

Tom Gallagher is an internist by training, but he has found his niche in CRPs (Communication and Resolution Programs). CRPs are intended to resolve medical error and adverse-event issues quickly and fairly, and they strive to address the needs of all parties involved—patients, families, doctors, nurses, administrators. For example, many medical professionals feel awkward talking to patients about errors, and conversely many patients don't feel comfortable confronting their doctors. CRPs assist in the communication process and also conduct a prompt investigation into the event. Providing timely information for patients is an important goal, as is tending to emotional fallout on all sides. CRPs are committed to a constructive response, helping the institution develop a plan to prevent such errors in the future. CRPs can even help negotiate financial settlements. Done right, CRPs would avoid the foot-dragging pace (and adversarial poison) of malpractice suits and help fix the system along the way. Like the theoretical health courts, CRPs have the potential to help many more people than malpractice suits, since there is not such a steep barrier to entry.

Gallagher pointed out that CRPs aren't about letting doctors go scot-free, a common misconception. "Doctors should be accountable," he told me, "but they shouldn't be responsible for problems with the system." System failures are like traps, he said, that will sooner or later ensnare an otherwise conscientious staff member (and that person's patient). This could be an apt description of Dr. Bawa-Garba and Jack Adcock.

Gallagher spoke about the concept of a "just culture," where the response to an error depends on the context. If a nurse reached for an IV bag of lactated Ringer's solution but grabbed a bag of saline by mistake, the hospital shouldn't fire him. An accidental, unintentional error like that is part of the human condition. The appropriate response—after addressing any harm to the patient—is to fix the storage system so that it's not possible to mix up the two types of IV bags. It would also be important to attend to the emotional response of the nurse, who might feel devastated that his split-second reach for the wrong bag might have harmed his patient.

Other errors, however, stem from at-risk behavior. For example, many doctors take shortcuts when writing notes in the EMR by doing a "cut-and-paste" from a previous note. In doing this, a doctor might miss a patient's renal insufficiency and so neglect to appropriately lower a medication dose. The appropriate response here—after addressing the harm to the patient—would be to educate the staff as to why cut-and-paste is a bad idea: you might squeak by 99% of the time, but it puts you at risk—*every* time—for making an error. It's also critical to take an honest look at a system that is so time-crunched that staff are forced to cut corners in order to keep up. A hospital would do well to proactively ask its doctors and nurses which shortcuts the system forces them to use; an avalanche of at-risk behaviors would likely come to light.

Then there are errors that result from out-and-out recklessness, such as a surgeon showing up to the OR drunk or a doctor knowingly ignoring standards of care. Even if no harm comes to the patient—as in the case of Dr. Simon Bramhall, who lasered his initials onto his patients' livers—true negligence requires disciplinary action. A lawsuit might be part of that action. (And even though the individual is held fully responsible for this negligence, it is still worth examining the system for exacerbating causes. A culture of hierarchy and impunity, for example, might enable someone like Dr. Bramhall to consider his act as "harmless." A high rate of burnout and substance abuse, for example, could reflect a punishing work environment or low morale. These situations are toxic for both staff and patients.)

The basis of CRPs is fairness. Patients should be treated fairly and so should medical staff. Like the Patient Compensation System in Denmark, CRPs would allow many more patients to have their cases addressed. In contrast to the Danish system (or the health courts), though, CRPs pledge to offer compensation comparable to what a patient might achieve with a court settlement. This is part of the "fairness" principle.

A hospital accountant might cast a jaundiced eye upon such fairness. If CRPs allow more patients to have their cases considered *and* offer settlements comparable to the court system, a hospital could be shelling out a lot more money to a lot more patients. A hospital might prefer to take the risks with good old-fashioned lawsuits, since so few patients are able to access the system, and even when they do, they usually lose. From a hard-nosed budgetary angle, CRPs might seem like a losing proposition.

Michelle Mello—the legal scholar who has written about health courts—researched this very question. She and her colleagues studied four hospitals in Boston that implemented CRPs. They calculated how much money each hospital had to pay out in liability costs over the first four years of the program and compared it to the four years before the program started. They also compared this to four similar hospitals that did not use CRPs. Their overall conclusion was that CRPs did not cost the hospitals more money, and in fact the number of lawsuits went down.[2] They suspected that open and forthright discussion about adverse events with patients causes fewer of them to file claims. This makes sense given that many people—like Nancy and Melissa—file lawsuits precisely because they cannot obtain information about what happened.

The tenets of the CRPs were appealing to Nancy—particularly the focus on direct communication with patients and families—and she offered to use some of her settlement money to help fund CRP training in Kansas. Tom Gallagher was game, and five years after Glenn's death the first CRP training session was held in the Sunflower State. It was a modest affair, with representatives from twenty local hospitals in attendance, mostly midlevel administrators. Melissa stood up first, thanked the audience for attending, and explained how the conference had come to be. Her presentation style is Midwestern straightforward, reliably unpretentious, but still she choked up when describing how her father had not been promptly transferred to a burn center and how he died eleven days later. She nevertheless soldiered on and spent thirty minutes walking the audience through her family's journey to learn what had transpired in her father's care.

"That's what happened," she said flatly, after concluding her thirty-third slide documenting phone calls, letters, inquiries, requests for information, and hours of deposition. "But here's what *should have* happened," she quickly followed up. "As soon as the local hospital learned from the burn center that the transfer should have occurred immediately, they should have reached out to my family."

Melissa laid out an unambiguous plan of action. "They should have let us know they were aware of this and that they were going to investigate. And in a few weeks they should have gotten back to us and told us, 'Here's what we learned. Here's why this happened. And here are the steps we're taking so that this doesn't happen again.'

"Had they done that," Melissa continued, "it would have let us know that they realized they'd screwed up. It would have communicated that they were taking their responsibilities seriously and that they had a level of integrity. Had they done that . . ." Here Melissa paused, and the exhaustion of the years'-long journey was evident as she gestured toward her data-packed slides on the screen, "*none* of this would have happened."

Nancy took the podium next. Her first slide was a portrait of Glenn. It was a school-photo type of portrait, showing a smiling, avuncular man in a brown jacket and tie. He looks like an approachable principal, the kind of school administrator whose door is always open.

In Nancy's presentation, she reconstructed the details of Glenn's medical care, the details that had taken years of painstaking effort to extract. She delivered her presentation in the subdued, no-nonsense voice of the fourth-grade teacher that she was. But her voice faltered when she got to the end, where the burn center doctors recommended that she discontinue life support. "That was the hardest decision of my life," she said, her words barely audible above the emotion. "He died within five minutes." The room hushed.

Nancy's final slide brought back the portrait of Glenn. His presence seemed to give her courage to continue. "Using hindsight," she said, her voice gathering strength and then blossoming into anger, "I wished I'd *raised hell* when that doctor put Glenn into the ICU." Her words reverberated across the room, with exactly the forcefulness and shock you might experience upon hearing your fourth-grade teacher let loose an expletive.

She persevered through the rest of her presentation, her voice taut with determination and pain. Nancy stood next to the portrait of her beloved husband of forty-six years and concluded with a simple statement: "I now know what happened. But the one question I never got an answer to is, 'Why?'"

# CHAPTER FOURTEEN

# BRINGING ALONG
# OUR BRAINS

"You can't nail jelly to a tree."

This was how Itiel Dror, a cognitive neuroscientist, described to me the challenges of changing a culture. In this case we were talking about the medical culture, especially as it relates to fixing medical error. Things such as hierarchy, communication style, traditions of training, work ethic, egos, socialization, professional ideals—these are all deeply ingrained in the culture and have roles in both committing and preventing errors.

Moreover, there is the broader culture within which the medical community dwells. The United States, for example, has a zealous tradition of individualism. It's also comfortably litigious. European countries, by and large, are more willing to place limits on what individuals can pursue, both in terms of medical care and litigation of errors. Trying to remake these cultures, even with the noble intention of decreasing medical errors, is futile. Like nailing jelly to a tree.

Every country and every hospital is saturated with layers of existing rules—written and unwritten—governed by money, by liability, and by regulatory bodies. Dror recognizes that a sea change in the current system isn't coming soon. Making little tweaks within the current difficult system is the best we can do.

But Dror has a big beef with our typical approach to tweaking the medical system. Each time we train the hospital staff to address one type of error, it's very likely that much of the instruction will be forgotten in a few months. Each time we set up yet another checklist in the electronic medical record, it's very likely that most of the staff will soon tune it out. Plaster the hallways with cognitively ineffective posters, touting the latest quality-improvement initiative, and there's no doubt that they'll fade into the background blur within weeks.

"The problem," Dror says, "is that these methods are not brain friendly." He illustrates this point with the example of passwords. As a typical hospital employee, I have passwords for the EMR, for my desktop computer, for the hospital email, for the medical school email, for the statewide prescription drug database, for the appointment system, for the on-call system, for the X-ray viewing system, and for the EKG viewing system.

And those are just the passwords medical workers use every day for work. We all have another dozen or so personal passwords that clog our brains. These passwords change every three to six months and each have exacting— and exactingly different—requirements for capital letters, numerals, special characters, and the genomic analysis of your pet gerbil. Furthermore, we are exhorted by whippersnappers in the IT department who are hardly old enough to vote to *never* use the same password twice. And *never ever ever ever* write your passwords down.

"That policy looks good on paper," Dror said, "but it doesn't take into account the human element, the way our brains really work." As one who repeats passwords ad infinitum and who secretly writes all of them down (okay, in an undisclosed location, but still), I was exceedingly relieved to hear this. "You don't have to be a cognitive neuroscientist," he said, "to know that people *have* to write their passwords down and/or use the same password on various systems."

There are countless examples in medicine of things that are the precise opposite of brain friendly. In one iteration of our EMR, for example, there was a particular spot in the note where the doctor was asked yes/no questions for two different screening issues. In one instance, you had to press 1 or 2 to indicate "yes" or "no." In the other you had to press Y or N to indicate "yes" or "no." It's a minuscule point, but it drove me bonkers each and every %$@# time. I felt almost embarrassed getting upset over such a small thing, but it never failed to get my goat.

Talking to Dror made me understand why: the EMR setup lacked cognitive consistency. My trusty brain is always searching for efficiency, and so it wasted no time "thinking" when I came to that first yes/no question—my fingers automatically reached for the number keys to choose 1 or 2. Of course I hit a wall when I did this at the next yes/no question, which required the Y and N keys. For me, it was just endless aggravation, but for Dror it's an unnecessary cognitive load and thus a potential source of error. The EMR caused me to waste precious cognitive resources sorting out whether to head for the number keys or the letter keys. Given the finite capacities of our brains, this yes/no idiocy—which I was forced to suffer through for every single patient every single day—squandered some of my thinking ability. I thus had less of it available to think about my patients' actual medical conditions and less of it available to keep an eye out for errors.

A brain-friendly EMR would offer exactly one way of answering yes/no questions, and it would be consistent everywhere across the system, whether you are answering questions about your patients' latex allergies or their DNR status, or whether it's okay to substitute a generic for a brand-name medication, or whether you want to enlarge the font size because staring at the computer screen has annihilated the last vestiges of your visual cortex.

The yes/no function is just one microscopic cog in the system, but consider all the seemingly minute inconsistencies in the EMR and then all the inconsistencies of all the other myriad technologies in medicine (and hoo boy, don't get me started!), and they add up to a boatload of wasted brain reserve. All of which is directly subtracted from patient care. This is brainpower that we want focused on avoiding a medical error, not used for sorting through alerts for drug interactions with alcohol wipes, or pregnancy warnings for 70-year-olds, or ICU alarms that go off when a patient scratches his nose, or well-meaning tobacco screens that require the identical amount of documentation for the patient who quit 45 years ago as for the patient who currently smokes two packs a day, or the prescription field that insists that you distinguish between capsules and caplets, or the language screen that asks you to clarify whether you used a live interpreter or a phone interpreter right after you've typed in that both you and the patient speak English, or the Past Medical History screen that I had efficiently memorized as choice #18 but that was pushed up to #19 when some other choice was added so that now #18 brought up Past Obstetrical History, which I proceeded to add to every patient that first week only to learn that there was no possibility of deleting it, so now a whole cohort of my male patients all have their obstetrical histories dutifully and permanently noted in their medical records. But perhaps I digress . . .

"This doesn't just stress you and frustrate you," Dror said. "It depresses you." Truer words were never spoken. At the end of a ten-hour day battling these EMR inanities, it's not just that I'm drained. It's that it feels as though we're forced to machete our way through the EMR jungle just to get to the place where we can finally *begin* the medical care of our patients. If we even have any functioning neurons left.

There is a burgeoning field of research examining how the "toxic" work environment in healthcare is contributing to burnout among doctors and nurses. The demands of the EMR can't be blamed for all of this, to be sure, but most medical folks would say that it is certainly the heavy hitter. There is a growing sense that rather than these technologies helping us to serve our patients, the tables have been turned so that *we* have to serve the *technologies*. Patient care is shunted off to the side, a quaint leftover that is subservient to the primary goal of documentation.

As a child, Itiel Dror was fascinated by the story of Pinocchio. Having a mind necessitated a miracle, some sort of fairy dust. Frankenstein's monster, by contrast, was just a set of body parts constructed in a laboratory according to a scientific recipe. Growing up on three different continents—his professor parents juggled alternating sabbaticals—Dror was drawn to people watching. He was fascinated by what was tinkering inside their heads, the fairy dust that made them take all sorts of actions, even ones that could seem illogical or counterproductive. He initially studied philosophy but found himself intrigued by the courses he took in artificial intelligence, computer science, and psychology. Eventually he chose to do his PhD in cognitive neuroscience, as it seemed to strike a middle ground that intersected with all these subjects.

Itiel Dror isn't a medical doctor, but he's studied the medical environment enough to reach his conclusion that medical errors are absolutely inevitable. This is simply the nature of the system. In any given medical encounter, he points out, there is a sea of information—usually piecemeal in nature—and most often not enough time to properly wade through it all. On top of that, the human brain has finite resources and so is constantly prioritizing which information to attend to. The relentless time pressure combined with the high stakes of the situation place even greater demands on the brain, so this humble organ has had to develop all sorts of strategies to survive. It filters information, for example, paying attention to certain tidbits while ignoring the rest. It utilizes an assortment of automatic habits and shortcuts. It relies on a trove of previous experiences and a library of recognizable patterns. The brain has limited capacity and is continually honing mechanisms to make up for its shortcomings.

These are brilliant survival strategies, enabling us to achieve what would otherwise be impossible in the slender amounts of time clinicians typically have for decision-making. But the very mechanisms of the brain that allow for such snazzy cogitations also make it prone to error. The brain easily falls prey to pitfalls, such as tunnel vision, groupthink, overconfidence, and biases of all flavors.

People don't make mistakes only because they are stupid, Dror said. They also make mistakes because they are smart. (I found this oddly comforting, in a roundabout sort of way.) Smart brains develop shortcuts—that's what

enables these brains to handle so much information and still make their own-
ers sound intelligent. Shortcuts are not a side effect of intelligence; they are
actually the *basis* of intelligence. Viewed in that light, you could actually interpret some medical errors as side effects of being smart.

Medical errors, in Dror's opinion, are the "inevitable outcome" of our neu-
rocognitive system squashed into the demanding medical environment. This
is why he has concluded that it is impossible to eliminate them. Although
"eradicating" medical errors sounds good in a hospital mission statement or
on a grant application, it's fundamentally impossible given the realities of our
brains and the nature of healthcare.

Humans utilize two predominant modes of thinking, often called simply
"fast" and "slow." Fast thinking is what we do in the moment; it is experiential.
Slow thinking is more analytical. Most training tools are geared toward slow,
analytical thinking (a new set of rules to memorize, another online module to
complete, another checklist to fill out, yet another training session to endure).
But most of what we actually do in medicine is in the moment. It's nearly all
fast, experiential thinking, so all that lumbering preparatory work is wasted.
It's nailing jelly to a tree.

Dror argues that we need to tailor any improvements we propose for reducing medical error to how the brain *actually* works. Rather than chasing the
impossible idealized goal of eliminating medical error, his research focuses on
error mitigation. Since you can't get rid of all the errors, you can work to make
the errors less damaging. The goal is rapid error *recognition* and even faster error *recovery*—all things that happen in the moment.[1]

Focusing on error recovery, rather than error prevention, is more effective because it is brain friendly. One example that Dror uses is handwashing.
Even though cleanliness edges out even godliness as the number-one way
to reduce hospital infections, medical personnel are embarrassingly lax with
their ablutions. In my hospital, as in every other hospital, there are posters
and signs and buttons affixed to every available surface exhorting handwashing. All of these earnestly laminated efforts, Dror says, are predominantly a
waste of time; our brains quickly relegate them to background noise in an
effort to focus their finite capacities on more pressing things. But what if the
senior doctor marched into the ICU—sans washing—with her entire medical
team in tow? Then, just before her stethoscope breached the patient's gown,
she stopped and turned to the team—with appropriately dramatic flair—and
asked, "Did anyone notice anything wrong?" After the error is identified and
discussed, she could ask the even more important question: "Why didn't any
of you speak up when you noticed that I didn't wash my hands?"

Dror calls his technique the "Terror of Error," and it is based on using these sorts of unpleasant but ultimately memorable experiences. Especially the squirmy discomfort of if/how/when to confront a superior. The emotional content keys into a different cognitive pathway than do the endless hand-washing signs plastered in the hallway. Once an emotional component is tied into an experience, it is remembered much more intensely and intuitively.

When I was an intern I once had to perform a physical exam on a patient in front of an attending for an end-of-rotation evaluation. In my nervousness or my hurry, I neglected to wash my hands. When the attending pointed that out—in front of the patient—I was mortified. My cheeks bloomed red as I shamefacedly edged over to the sink and slathered a gallon of antibacterial soap on my hands. But I never forgot that experience—the Terror of Error. Decades later, I can remember the exact room, the exact attending, the exact diagnosis of the patient, and of course, the painfully accrued lesson in handwashing. My current patients probably think I have obsessive-compulsive disorder as I wash and rewash my hands before and after—and sometimes during—the slightest physical contact. Public humiliation is not a recommended pedagogical strategy, of course, but it does point out the power of a lesson that is entwined with emotion. Not to mention the critical need for having hand-lotion dispensers parked next to every sink.

Experiencing failure on a personal level sticks with us in a way that recited rules can never do. It creates an emotional representation that worms into the depths of our brains. This may, in fact, be evolutionary. Imagine that news of distant coyote attacks has reached a hunter-gatherer society in the Paleolithic era. The leaders of this society might try to prevent attacks by warning its members to "Be Aware!" and "Stay Safe!" They might rally community members to aspire to "A Culture of Safety." They might remind people, "If you see something, say something." But the average hunter-gatherers are focusing their finite cognitive resources on, well, hunting and gathering. They will quickly tune out these exhortations, no matter how snappy or how focus-group-honed the phrasing is.

But when the first baby is snatched by a coyote—everything changes. This emotionally charged experience is processed in a different part of the brain than the anodyne warnings are. The realness of the experience by necessity carries much more weight in terms of survival, and may be why this cognitive strategy has been evolutionarily successful.

Luckily for us, though, realness doesn't actually have to be real to be effective. In airline security, for example, we need the baggage screeners to be alert for bombs and weapons. The "Stay Alert" signs that are posted everywhere may as well be abstract art for the staff who toil there day in and day out. Pass a few fake bombs through security, though, and you will get people's attention in a way that sticks in the brain.

Errors make sense when you understand the cognitive shortcuts that lead to them, and that's what Dror tries to teach nurses and doctors. When he helps hospitals set up simulation programs, he makes sure the staff get to experience errors. Instead of having the patient ultimately survive—as is the usual case in most simulations—Dror's exercises make sure the patient dies a few times. With high-stakes situations such as sepsis, cardiac arrest, intubation, surgical mistakes, and medication errors, it is important for the participants to experience things going wrong as a result of their decisions and actions. The experiential aspect of the training offers the strongest chance of transferring the knowledge to situations with real patients.

Simulation is preferred because personal experience with such disasters might actually be too traumatic to be effective. I remember when I was a resident and botched a case of diabetic ketoacidosis, nearly putting the patient into cardiac arrest. I was only a few days out of internship and was so devastated by the experience that I could hardly scrape my sorry self off the linoleum floor, much less think analytically about what had transpired and how to do better the next time. So I appreciated Dror's preference for simulation over personal experience. It wouldn't be a stretch to assume that patients also prefer simulation as the place for medical staff to experience the Terror of Error.

Dror pointed out a few other reasons why personal experience might not be the most effective vehicle for teaching. Often these situations involve a rare case or a fluke, things that are not necessarily generalizable. Plus, people tend to overcompensate based on personal experience, especially if it was a particularly devastating event. In simulation, you can—as Dror delicately puts it—"calibrate the trauma" and then debrief afterward to make sure it's a constructive experience rather than a destructive one.

It is also critical to do training in groups rather than as individuals. For one thing, so much of medicine is practiced as a team in real life, and so many errors relate to communication among team members. There is also the reality that medical information is typically scattered among the members of teams—the nurse knows the vital signs, the intern knows the CT result, the attending knows the patient's past medical history, the physical therapist knows where the patient is weakest. So teaching error mitigation in groups jibes better with reality. Additionally, group settings allow individuals to engage in the far more approachable task of identifying errors in other people before turning the unsparing lens on yourself.

A training session might be set up to teach the management of low blood pressure in the ICU. A team of doctors and nurses is given a simulation of a patient with hypotension. Each person possesses some bits of information about the patient, and together they have to figure out how to manage the hypotension and keep the kidneys and brain in good working order without flooding the lungs or causing cardiac arrythmia.

Such simulations quickly feel real to the participants, especially if one of the team members is really part of the training staff, discreetly contributing errors to the process (suggesting a medication that the patient is allergic to, mixing up buttons on the IV machine, forgetting some basic protocols, talking to the wrong person for the wrong thing). The training setup could involve rearranging equipment so that things aren't in their usual places. There could be real-world distractions—team members getting paged, phones ringing, a staff member heating up pungent fish stew in a nearby microwave. The team could be short-staffed because a nurse was pulled to cover for another team because *their* nurse was out sick. A critical medication could be on back order. The patient might speak Spanish, but admin sent over a Serbian translator. There could be a fire drill. The EMR could be temporarily unavailable because of routine maintenance—but your patience is greatly appreciated.

Dror advocates using such "sabotage" techniques because they create controlled errors. These sabotages heighten the experience of the errors in a constructive way, especially if the case ends in disaster. And of course, these sabotages mimic what happens in real life, so they are practical training. The real bonus, though, is that these sabotage-induced errors are much less fraught for team members to identify and analyze in the post-training discussion. After they are warmed up with these less threatening errors, they can segue into the more unsettling task of identifying their own errors and shortcomings.

This is particularly powerful in the realm of communication. We are told, ad infinitum, that poor communication causes errors. But hectoring doctors and nurses to "Communicate Well!" is about as effective as reiterating that advice to your toddlers (or your teenagers, or your hamsters). If the patient begins to slip away, however, as a result of communication errors in the exercise, the point is driven home in a way that resonates, and the situation can be analyzed with more meaning afterward.

Learning is even more powerful when it's unexpected. For example, the hypotension training exercise might be billed as a lesson about blood pressure management when in fact it was designed to teach about sepsis. If the session had been titled "Sepsis Training," everyone would have been in a sepsis state of mind, and there wouldn't be any learning about the *recognition* of sepsis, which—as we've seen—can be challenging.

Similarly, if a training session was titled "Communication Training," there would be so much "please," "pardon me," and "thank you" that it would feel like high tea with the Queen. We are, after all, diligently trained to produce what we think the person grading us wants to hear. Better to make it a training session about asthma management, but then weave in errors that arise from poor communication.

Most crucially, such training sessions should *never* be titled "Fixing Medical Error." It's hard to imagine a label that would more perfectly encourage participants to check the boxes they know the corporate-compliance supervisors need them to check off. Instead, these training sessions should be integrated seamlessly into the regular curriculum about treating cardiac arrest or adrenal insufficiency or acute psychosis, so that error issues are simply part of learning about the topic.

When the staff members uncover the lessons experientially—figuring out how to rally a disorganized team or how to deal with missing equipment—the message sticks. The focus isn't on preventing errors per se, but rather on identifying and fixing them as they happen. Being forced to deal with errors in real time as the (simulated) patient is crashing is the epitome of what Itiel Dror sees as brain-friendly training. Contrast this to our typical way of teaching medicine: a lecture hall darkened to planetarium black, a light-year's worth of PowerPoint slides in rapid succession, each with eighty-seven bullet points in subatomic font accompanied by a series of inscrutable graphs and an apologetic mono-toned speaker saying, "I know this is hard to read, but . . ." It's hard to conceive of anything less brain friendly for learners. You might as well distribute a tab of Valium to every audience member in the first minute of the session—teddy bear and goose-down quilt optional—and call it a day. The learning retention would be about the same, though you'd probably get better course evaluations at the end.

Simulations can be startlingly realistic. On a warm spring day, I found myself doing an unusual set of medical rounds in one of Bellevue's towering brick behemoths that date from 1905. The ward had come full circle over the course of a century. After caring for generations of New York City's sickest, it had been demoted to offices and storage units when the new hospital building was erected. But now it was back as a ward, with fully functioning medical rooms and bustling staff in scrubs and white coats. The patients were still genuine salt-of-the-earth New Yorkers but with perhaps a bit more avid Stanislavski training.

Peering through a one-way mirror I watched a patient fidget in his cotton gown that dangled open at back. A hacking cough erupted periodically. His partner paced the room anxiously, occasionally dropping into the bedside chair and leaning in toward the bed. The two men clasped and unclasped hands, attempting to steady each other. The patient's pneumonia had not improved, despite antibiotics. The chest X-ray showed a rising tide of fluid accumulating around the lung. If that fluid was merely a reaction to the pneumonia, it would likely resolve on its own. But if that fluid were infected—an empyema—the patient would need a large-bore chest tube inserted by a surgeon to drain it. And maybe the pneumonia was masking a lung cancer, and the fluid was harboring malignant cells.

In order to distinguish between these possibilities, the doctors needed to perform a bedside thoracentesis to sample the fluid. They'd pass a medium-size needle through the back muscles just far enough to access the fluid but (hopefully!) not so far as to puncture the lung. But first, they'd need to obtain informed consent. This being an academic medical center, the lowly medical student was dispatched to do the task.

Wearing a short white coat over her scrubs and white-knuckling a clipboard to her chest, the medical student explained the situation and the reason for the thoracentesis. The patient and his partner visibly blanched as she enumerated the possible risks of collapsed lung, internal bleeding, and spreading of the infection. The student herself blanched under the weight of the awful outcomes she was describing. She seemed as unsettled as the patient at the prospect of a needle transgressing some of the body's most crucial organs. She tried not to unduly terrify the patient, but that didn't seem possible. The patient and his partner wavered between tentative reassurance and wild-eyed panic, peppering the student with questions she couldn't always answer about a procedure she'd never actually performed.

In the next three rooms, three other medical students were bumbling simultaneously through the same agonies of informed consent with three other pneumonia patients and their anxious partners.

In four rooms farther down the hall, medical students struggled to figure out what to do for a post-op patient who'd ceased to produce urine, while a scrub-clad nurse waited impatiently for an answer. Was this a harbinger of full-on renal failure? Was the patient about to go south, fast? On the other side of the hall were four rooms of medical students grappling with a case of sky-high blood pressure in a patient who also complained of a headache. Was the headache a distraction or was it a sign of an impending intracranial bleed? The patients were fake, but the pressure on the students was real.

These medical students were about to graduate and become interns with certifiable MDs after their names. They were participating in the aptly titled "First Night on Call" exercise, a simulation program developed by a team of educators led by my NYU colleagues Adina Kalet and Sondra Zabar. The students have ten minutes to handle these tense clinical situations—created by remarkably convincing actors—and then they have to present the cases to (real) chief residents or attending physicians to be grilled on the clinical details. After that, the students engage in what many feel is the most valuable part—a group discussion analyzing their experiences in the simulation. A faculty member facilitates the discussion, but it's the students who dig through the issues—medical, emotional, logistical, hierarchical—that are unearthed. The students consistently rank the simulation as one of the most effective learning experiences in medical school.

But are they effective in reducing medical error? This is an unwieldy question to study because it is exceedingly labor intensive to gather enough actors (and rooms and time and supervising faculty) to generate a sample size robust enough to detect a change in error rates—outcomes that are both uncommon and hard to detect. Nevertheless, there are some encouraging data.[2] Simulation training for procedures such as placing central lines, intubating patients, and doing colonoscopies showed benefits for patients, such as fewer central line infections and higher rates of successful intubation or colonoscopy. Procedures are obviously much easier to study than doing adequate informed consent or figuring out why urine production has ceased, but simulation holds promise as a way to improve patient safety without patients having to suffer the learning curve.

When I observed the sessions, it was remarkable how real they seemed. The actors did not let up on the students, not for one second, asking difficult questions, sputtering with cough, welling up with emotion. Even though they knew it was a simulation, the students told me that once they were in the room, it felt entirely like a real episode on call.

The only notable difference from a real night on call at Bellevue was that while the students were off with their attendings, the actors used their break time to compare notes in a back room about their various auditions and theater productions. The day that I observed, two actors—one wearing a patient's gown and the other wearing nurses' scrubs—figured out that they'd both been in *A Chorus Line*, though at different times. Without missing a beat, they launched into a perfectly executed Broadway number. The patient's gown wasn't fully tied at the back, so it billowed out like a spinnaker on the crisp pirouettes and step-ball-change moves. When the two dancers snapped to a meticulously coordinated end, which elicited applause from the onlookers, the gown wafted languidly down, obediently returning to its standard-issue sag.

Come to think of it, something like this probably *has* happened at some point on the wards of Bellevue.

As I've discussed earlier, technology has the ability to cause many errors. But of course it has the potential to prevent errors, which is why most of this technology was developed in the first place. From Itiel Dror's perspective, the key is to design technology with a knowledge of our cognitive limitations. The goal is to tinker with the system—rather than with the humans—to make things safer. The technology doesn't have to be overly complex to minimize errors, but it does need to be brain friendly. This can often be accomplished with basic nuts and bolts. In the operating room, for example, anesthesiologists have access to oxygen and nitrogen. In the past, patients have died when the wrong gas was administered. The gas tanks were color-coded to prevent this, but every year there were still a few cases in which the hoses were mixed up. Finally someone thought to redesign the cheap little connectors and just make them two different sizes for the two different gases. Thereafter, it was physically impossible to connect a hose to the wrong gas.

Another fix along these cognitive lines is to standardize the way equipment is set up. For example, the crash cart—used for resuscitating patients in cardiac arrest—should be arranged in one way only, so that the correct medications can be found quickly, with less chance of mix-up. Better yet, the contents of the cart should be arranged in a brain-friendly way. In one study, researchers let pharmacists and nurses organize the setup of the crash cart in a way that made sense given how they used the medications in practice. When the new arrangement was tested against the standard setup, staff members were able to retrieve medications more quickly and more accurately.[3]

Other errors could be minimized by eliminating similar-sounding names of medications that our brains have trouble distinguishing. One doesn't have to plumb the etymological depths to imagine the possibilities for error with medications with names like Ditropan and Diprivan. You'd hate to accidentally treat someone's overactive bladder by knocking them unconscious with an intravenous anesthetic. Nor would you want to mix up Lunesta and Neulasta and give that poor insomniac a syringe full of bone-marrow activator.

There are more than a septillion words you can construct with the 26 letters of the English alphabet. Thus, there's no logical reason for Celexa, Celebrex, and Cerebyx to coexist in our pharmacologic universe, given that they treat depression, pain, and seizures, respectively. Ditto for Lamictal and Lamisil, unless you want to treat your seizures with anti-fungal cream.

And while we're at it, we should tackle the dangerous sound-alikes that have the additional bonus of being utterly unpronounceable. What Madison Avenue dream team, I'd like to know, came up with Farxiga and Fetzima?

They somehow made it possible to accidentally treat someone's diabetes with an antidepressant *and* give the doctor tendinitis of the tongue in the process. Sound-alike and difficult-to-pronounce medication names are perfect examples of the multitude of brain-*unfriendly* minutiae that clutter up modern medicine. Added up, they squander copious amounts of mental energy, energy that should be focused on patient care.

In order to minimize error and improve safety, we have to take into account the human element and then design systems and teaching methods that work with the realities of our gray matter. How our brains work doesn't usually make the top-ten list when healthcare concerns are prioritized. But it ought to. Otherwise we'll just keep nailing jelly to the tree.

# CHAPTER FIFTEEN

# THE RECKONING

When something goes wrong in a hospital, the traditional response is the morbidity and mortality conference (the M&M). This picks through the minutiae of the case, trying to home in on the specific errors in the medical care. A broader approach to error is something known as root cause analysis, which looks not just for what went wrong but also for what weaknesses in the system made it possible for things to go wrong (and of course how to prevent this in the future).

Jay's case exemplifies the fact that medical error is rarely just one specific thing. Instead—as also seen with Glenn and with Jack Adcock—most medical errors are the result of a cascade of actions that compound one another. Each of the small things, by themselves, might not cause a bad outcome, but together, they do.

To recap, Jay was a healthy 39-year-old man who was diagnosed with AML (acute myelogenous leukemia). He underwent his first round of chemotherapy (induction chemo) and had to be readmitted to the hospital a few days later with a fever and low white count (neutropenia). Over the course of three days, Jay grew progressively sicker. He was treated for MRSA blood infection but died of cardiopulmonary arrest.

"Please know," Tara wrote to me, "that I realize that AML with trisomy 11 involvement is not a walk in the park, and I am well aware that the statistics were not in Jay's favor. But the AML did not kill Jay; his poorly treated infection killed him."

So let's try to take apart the errors in Jay's case that added up to the tragic outcome. In thinking this through, I've come up with several concrete errors, specific actions that are relatively straightforward to evaluate, such as the decisions about removing the central line or transferring Jay to the ICU. And then there are errors that are less tangible to describe, those that are more about human interactions and the culture of the hospital. These are much harder to fit into neat algorithms, but they contribute just as much to medical error.

It's worth considering each of these errors in turn, because there is much that can be illuminated from each one. Moreover, these errors exemplify the relationship in medicine between the concrete aspects of care and the less tangible aspects. They also illuminate the challenges of *preventing* medical error: it's easy to make a checklist for how to evaluate a fever or rules for when to remove an indwelling catheter, but you can't checklist clinical thoroughness, good listening, effective communication, intellectual humility, or professional responsibility.


## THE VACUTAINER

Two days after Jay was discharged from his hospitalization for induction chemotherapy, he had his blood drawn in the doctor's office. The nurse drawing the blood struggled to get the Vacutainer to connect to his indwelling catheter. At one point, the Vacutainer fell onto the white paper of the exam table where Jay was sitting. The nurse picked it up, reattached it to the catheter, and proceeded to draw blood and then flush saline through the catheter.

Tara is convinced that the MRSA infection in Jay's bloodstream was caused by this action, that the Vacutainer became contaminated upon touching the exam table and then went on to contaminate the catheter. MRSA can live for days and even weeks outside the body, so this could be plausible. (MRSA has been found living on stethoscopes, scrubs, bedrails, and hospital curtains, and there have been documented outbreaks of infection related to these.) Of course, Tara's theory could not be proved unless that particular Vacutainer were to be cultured and then found to have the identical strain of MRSA present in Jay's bloodstream.

However, even if the Vacutainer were not the cause of the infection, what that nurse did was still an error. Once any blood-drawing apparatus falls onto an exam table, it should be discarded (or properly sterilized before use). For patients with impaired immune systems, this step is particularly important. Nurses who work with immunosuppressed patients should know better.

It's fairly clear, therefore, that the handling of the Vacutainer was an error, but it's not possible to tell if that nurse's action transmitted the MRSA infection to Jay's bloodstream. This incident emphasizes the point that the presence of an error and the presence of a bad outcome don't necessarily mean the two are linked. Furthermore, even if the incorrectly used Vacutainer did in fact transmit the MRSA infection, it would still be a stretch to say that this event was *the* cause of Jay's death. As with most medical errors, it usually takes many more missteps by many more people for an error to translate into a death.

## THE INDWELLING CATHETER

When I read through Jay's case the first time, I remember feeling a nervous itch in my fingers as his clinical course worsened. They kept wanting to jump onto the page and yank out that catheter. If there is one thing that is pummeled into the brains of interns during medical training, it's that as soon as *any* patient spikes a fever, all foreign bodies (central lines, urinary catheters, arterial lines) are immediate suspects. They all should be removed promptly unless there is a compelling reason not to do so.

For patients with suppressed immune systems like Jay's, the urgency is even greater. There has got to be a persuasive and well-articulated reason to leave in any foreign body when it comes to a neutropenic patient with a fever. For example, if there is absolutely no other IV access and loss of that catheter would mean the patient couldn't receive life-saving medications, the doctor might make the reluctant decision to leave in the catheter. But this was not the case. Tara commented, with no small amount of pride, that Jay had "marvelously gigantic venous access," which of course would be expected in a fit 39-year-old who'd never been sick before. One other possible reason to leave in a catheter is that an alternative source of the infection was clearly identified and treated (e.g., a urinary tract infection), but even then most doctors would remove the catheter to avoid the possibility of it being "seeded" by the urinary organisms—especially with a patient who is immunosuppressed.

However, there is not the slightest shade of gray once blood cultures show definitive evidence of bacteria. Neutropenia, fever, foreign bodies, and blood-borne bacteria are a volatile mix. The only element in that tinder box that can be instantly rectified is the removal of the foreign body.

Admittedly, once bacteria are noted in the blood culture, it can still take another 24 hours to identify the exact bug (which is crucial for selecting the right antibiotic). Furthermore, "positive blood cultures" can occasionally be a false alarm, with the culture revealing nonpathogenic bacteria that just happened to be along for the ride (referred to as contamination). But in a febrile patient who lacks a sufficient immune system, you can't wait the additional 24 hours to determine if it's merely a case of contamination—the stakes are too high. So the first whiff of "positive blood cultures" is generally a mandate to pull the line, *stat*.

Midday on that Sunday, two days before Jay died, a nurse told Jay of his blood cultures: "There's all sorts of stuff growing in there." It would be another

24 hours before the microbiology lab could identify the bacteria as MRSA. Finding multiple organisms in the culture—if that's indeed what the nurse was referring to—is more common in contamination, but it certainly doesn't rule out a true infection. Jay had just received chemotherapy, his immune system was shot, and he had been persistently febrile for 48 hours despite receiving broad-spectrum antibiotics. I cannot come up with a plausible reason to leave in the catheter.

Not only was the catheter not pulled; it was actively used during the ensuing 24 hours to administer fluids, transfusions, and antibiotics. If the catheter was indeed the source of infection, then using the line for 24 additional hours was simply infusing more bacteria into Jay's bloodstream.

The next day, the bacteria in the blood cultures were identified as MRSA—a true infection, not a contaminant. Staph aureus is a skin-dwelling organism, so a catheter piercing his skin and offering a toll-free highway directly to Jay's bloodstream would be the clear culprit. However, Jay's catheter couldn't be removed immediately because his platelets were dangerously low, so hemorrhage during the removal was a real risk. It took several more hours for Jay to receive sufficient platelet transfusion to allow for safe removal. One can quibble about the exact timing, but there's no doubt that the infected catheter remained in Jay's body longer than it should have.

## TRANSFERRING TO THE ICU

Why wasn't Jay transferred to the ICU? This question plagued me as I followed his progressive decline over the three days of his hospitalization. There were so many points where I thought, "Oh boy, this is where I'd be calling for help," or, "This is where I'd grab the gurney myself and wheel the patient over to the ICU." Admittedly, this partly reflects individual style. Every doctor and nurse develops his or her own clinical style, and one key requirement is knowing your own comfort level and being aware of your biases. I know that I tend to be conservative—medically, at least. I try, for example, to hold off on newly released medications until I see how the dust settles. The downside of my hesitancy is that my patients may miss out on some of the benefits that newer drugs offer, but hopefully I avoid some as-yet-unknown disasters. Other doctors view the benefits for their patients as far outweighing the risks and so prescribe these new meds as soon as they're out of the gate. It's not that one approach is right and the other is wrong—they're just two different styles of practicing medicine.

Dr. Mueller and Dr. Peterson might have higher tolerance for acute illness than I do because they practice in medical specialties—oncology and pulmonary medicine—that experience a higher proportion of critically ill patients. Or their behavior could simply reflect their overall style of practicing medicine, something that is neither right nor wrong, just individual temperament.

On the extreme end are doctors who fall into the cowboy category, who would view transferring a patient to the ICU as some sort of personal failure, intimating that they aren't macho enough to tough it out. Cowboy medicine has receded somewhat over the years, as tolerance for ego-driven alpha doctors has waned. If anything, I observe that medical teams these days have swung the pendulum in the other direction—calling extra consults when they don't really need them, or pushing to transfer a patient to the ICU because they are afraid to care for a moderately sick patient on the regular ward. Usually this is from a risk-averse style of practice combined with a fear of a malpractice suit (though occasionally it's due to laziness). Without having personally spoken to any of Jay's physicians, I can't know the reasoning behind their reticence to transfer him to the ICU. They may well have had valid clinical reasons. Nevertheless, I found it striking that the team allowed a progressively decompensating patient to stay on the ward when ICU care was available within the hospital. (In hospitals without on-site ICUs, one has to weigh the additional risks of transferring an unstable patient via ambulance or helicopter.)

In my experience, though, this is where the nurse stands up and declares, "This patient needs to leave my floor ASAP and go to the ICU." Nurses are quite clear about the scope of medicine that can be handled in their particular clinical setting (ward, ER, step-down unit, CCU, etc.) and are usually reliably vocal when that scope is exceeded. For better or for worse, nurses usually err on the side of caution much more than doctors do. The critique of this, if any, is that some nurses adhere to an overly rigid interpretation of scope of care, and any patient who drifts even a hair's breadth beyond that is bundled up and transferred before you've even unfurled the stethoscope from your pocket. Thus, the absence of nurses rallying to get Jay moved was quite surprising to me.

It's true that some floor nurses aren't comfortable confronting doctors (though a healthy hospital environment should encourage such back-and-forth), but they would surely alert their supervisor if they felt that they were in over their head with a patient. The head nurse is responsible for ensuring that there is enough nursing power on the unit to handle all the patients and cannot afford to have a single patient sucking up excessive nursing resources. It is often on staffing grounds alone that the head nurse will insist that a critically ill patient be transferred immediately to the ICU.

The first hematology fellow—Dr. Amir—thought Jay might have had ARDS (acute respiratory distress syndrome) after he ordered an arterial blood gas in the early hours of Tuesday morning. His speculation may not have been borne out by the CT scan done later that day, but ARDS is one of those five-alarm-fire words that nurses do not take lightly. If a head nurse hears "ARDS" from one of the docs—even a junior one—she is usually pressing the attending physician to get the patient moved yesterday. (As a side note, it's worth pointing out that the typical X-ray and CT signs of ARDS may be absent in immunosuppressed patients. The black-and-white shadows that radiologists pick out as "abnormal" are a result of inflammation. If your white blood cells have been pulverized by chemotherapy, you are not able to mount the classic inflammatory response, so you could have ARDS despite "negative" scans.)

Looking at all of this together, what seemed to be lacking was a sense of urgency. The best that I could ascertain—admittedly from a secondhand source—was that Jay's steadily worsening condition did not light a fire under anyone. The doctors did not appear to be reacting aggressively, nor did any of the nurses seem to raise an alarm on either clinical or staffing grounds. Was this from lack of awareness? Lack of knowledge? Lack of "big picture" thinking? Lack of time to analyze all the data points? I recognize that I have the unfair benefit of 20/20 hindsight, but I still find the lack of reaction concerning.

After Jay's death, Tara learned an unusual fact about the bone marrow transplant unit in that hospital. It was a privatized unit. That is, the BMTU functioned almost like a separate hospital within the hospital. So a patient couldn't simply be "transferred" to the ICU but had to be formally discharged from the BMTU (as though the patient were going home) and then readmitted to the ICU as if a brand-new patient.

Seems like a lot of extra paperwork, especially if all you are doing is wheeling a patient from one floor to another. Why would a hospital privatize one of its units and add all these extra bureaucratic hurdles? The nursing staff of the BMTU, Tara learned, all worked for an outside agency. Why would the hospital contract out the nursing services rather than use its own nurses?

I'll admit I'm probably a bit cynical here, but when it comes to managerial rearrangements within the medical system, the reason is usually (though admittedly not always) money. Hospitals are always scrounging for cash, and some hit upon the novelty of privatizing certain services, often those that are already relatively self-contained. For example, radiology units typically exist in their own world within the hospital. Patients who need these services go there only for a brief period of time before returning to their home base (the medical ward, the surgical ward, etc.). Radiology is also an extremely expensive service to run because of the high-end technology.

Private companies saw an opportunity—they could set up private radiology units in multiple hospitals and pool radiologists to read the scans. The radiologists didn't even need to be on-site; they could read the scans from home. Or they could read them from Estonia, where they would cost less to hire. For individual hospitals, contracting such a service might be cheaper than running the units and hiring the staff themselves. For the private companies, they can turn a profit by pooling services and even equipment. It seems like a win-win, at least financially.

I remember the first time I came across a setup like that. The rehab service in our hospital functioned like its own hospital, even though it wasn't privately contracted. It always rubbed me the wrong way. First of all, it was a pain in the neck. Transferring a patient to any other service—surgery, geriatrics, OB-GYN—simply involved conferring with the respective teams and then wheeling the patient over. With rehab, though, you had to go through the entire discharge process—endless forms and busywork that fell on the shoulders of already overworked medical teams. The patient was only moving down to the fourth floor, but the paperwork needed for the transfer was the same as if it were for a full discharge from the hospital.

But even more than the logistical annoyances, something about this arrangement felt wrong to me philosophically. We are one hospital, right? All the different services—obstetrics, pediatrics, emergency medicine, neurology, internal medicine, oncology, psychiatry, surgery, radiology, anesthesiology, geriatrics, intensive care, ophthalmology, urology, neurosurgery, pharmacy, dialysis, laboratories—are critical facets of this larger and meaningful institution that we call a hospital. Even though some services (interventional cardiology) may bring in more revenue than others (gynecology), we are all part of this enterprise devoted to meeting the full spectrum of our patients' medical needs. It feels plain wrong to me that some parts are cordoned off.

So when trying to figure out why Jay wasn't transferred to the ICU as his condition steadily worsened, it crossed my mind—and Tara's too—that there might have been competing interests at play. (Glenn's wife, Nancy, entertained similar thoughts as she tried to figure out why her husband wasn't promptly transferred to the burn center.) "Discharging" Jay from the BMTU would have meant losing the revenue generated by his admission. He'd now be in the regular hospital, which would take over the billing and the revenue.

As much as I try, though, I can't bring myself to believe that money would drive the decision. I might be a bleeding-heart idealist, but I find it wholly impossible to imagine any doctor standing in front of a crashing patient and doing a calculation about revenue losses. Yes, I know that doctors can be as small-minded, greedy, selfish, vain, narcissistic (shall I go on?) as anyone else out there. But there is a baseline clinical instinct below which I cannot see any doctor or nurse falling: when a patient is acutely decompensating before you,

you are not thinking about money. I would find it hard—and heartbreaking—to believe that financial issues could trump clinical acuity in the moment.

However, subtle pressures should not be underestimated. I wonder if the staff at the BMTU had been given the message from higher-ups that discharges to the ICU should be avoided unless absolutely necessary. Or they might have been informed that the BMTU budget was under severe strain, that staff might be laid off and raises deferred. Staff might be urged to improve documentation to appropriately capture the severity of their patients' conditions (sicker patients merit higher payments). They might be reminded that the BMTU is a "comprehensive" unit that takes care of its patients at all levels of clinical need. They might be exhorted to "carefully consider the appropriateness" before discharging a patient to the ICU. Subtle pressures can be quite powerful. (If they weren't, you wouldn't see pharmaceutical sales reps showering doctors with pens, mugs, and sushi lunches.)

And even if financial issues—overt or subtle—didn't get in the way of transferring patients from the BMTU to the ICU, the logistical issues certainly might have. Discharging a patient involves a lot of paperwork, especially for nurses, and it's easy to imagine this as a disincentive to transfer.

About a year after Jay's death, Tara was taking a weekend workshop in critical-care nursing (all nurses are required to maintain certification with continuing education programs). During the break, she noticed a nurse wearing a sweatshirt with the logo of the hospital where Jay had been. Not mentioning her own experience, Tara began chatting with this ICU nurse. The lecture they'd just attended had been about septic shock, so the conversation flowed effortlessly toward commiserating about hypothetical patients with neutropenic fever and sepsis, and how they always got transferred to the ICU too late.

"The patients who come to our ICU," the nurse said, inhaling deeply from her cigarette, "don't have a chance in hell." She gave a sardonic laugh. "It takes forever to get these patients transferred to the ICU because we have a BMTU." ("Oh really?" Tara inquired.) "They can't come straight to the ICU," the nurse explained, "because they have to be completely readmitted like a new patient. By the time they actually get to the ICU, they're too far gone." Tara asked if she ever reported these concerns to her manager. The nurse just rolled her eyes and then took another magnificent drag on her cigarette.

So far, we've reviewed three concrete issues in Jay's care—reusing a Vacutainer that had fallen down, the delay in removing the indwelling catheter, and the reluctance to transfer Jay to the ICU. I'm going to assume there was no premeditated malice involved. Despite the jaded observations of this one ICU nurse, I honestly do not think that an entire oncology team thought, "Hmmm, we have this critically ill patient here. Let's *not* transfer him to the ICU." (Though there may have been subtle pressures at work.) To me, the real error was that it seems as though the staff simply did not recognize—or take seriously—how critically ill Jay was. This brings up the second category of errors, the ones that are less tangible.

### POOR CLINICAL EVALUATION

The first time I walked through the case with Tara, I tried hard not to assume the easy self-righteousness of a Monday-morning clinical quarterback. But it was hard to restrain myself as I watched a textbook case of sepsis unfold.

Sepsis is one of those paradoxical medical situations in which the body's protective mechanisms backfire and end up harming the patient. In response to an infection, the body normally unleashes a cascade of infection-fighting compounds. In the vast majority of cases, these do the trick and the infection is quashed. But occasionally this cascade can take on a life of its own, causing overwhelming inflammation that wreaks havoc on the body. Even with antibiotics to eradicate the bacteria, sepsis can power forward independently, leading to multisystem organ failure, as happened with Jay.

While sepsis can occur in anyone, it's more likely in patients who either have a handicapping susceptibility or have the bad luck of getting infected with a virulent organism. Jay had the misfortune of both. And once he had a fever, the conditions were ripe for sepsis. While it is possible to have fevers from causes other than infection, it is standard medical practice to consider fever as an infection until proven otherwise. When Jay spiked a fever after his initial chemotherapy, his medical team did the right thing—admitted him to the hospital and started broad-spectrum intravenous antibiotics, along with antifungal and antiviral agents. (He'd been on oral versions of these medications while he was home, but now he needed stronger doses.)

The initial clinical evaluation of a febrile patient is critical. Since the identity of the pathogen is unknown at the outset, the clinical evaluation is akin to detective work. Urinary burning would suggest a genito-urinary source. Neurologic impairment or mental-status changes might suggest meningitis or encephalitis. Nausea, vomiting, diarrhea, or abdominal pain could suggest a gastrointestinal source, though these symptoms can appear, nonspecifically, in infections from other sources.

A good clinical history ferrets out the minute details that could suggest which microbes might be wreaking the havoc: where you grew up, what kind of job you have, who's sick at home, whether you breed parrots, whether you've recently traveled to the tropics or been on the hajj, whether you've been hiking in the woods, whether you garden or keep an aquarium, whether you were recently hospitalized or incarcerated, whether you've been living in a nursing home or a college dormitory or a homeless shelter, whether you've had all your vaccinations, what medications you take, what illicit drugs you might have used, whom you've had sex with and whom *they've* had sex with.

A careful physical exam is also critical. A heart murmur could suggest infection of the heart valves (endocarditis). Abnormal breath sounds could suggest pneumonia. Joint swelling, swollen lymph nodes, characteristic rashes, enlarged spleen—these can all suggest particular types of infections.

I don't know how thorough a clinical evaluation Jay was given on admission. I've certainly seen some doctors squeak by with the most cursory of evaluations. One attending I witnessed when I was a student used to plunk his stethoscope in the midpoint of the patient's torso, taking in the cardiac sounds, breath sounds, and abdominal sounds all in one substandard listen. At the other end of the spectrum was the legendary Dr. Vincent McAuliffe, an infectious-disease attending who worked at Bellevue during the early years of the AIDS crisis.

One time when I was a resident, I found myself struggling with a complicated patient at 11 p.m. on a Friday. My attending had long since departed the hospital. I was alone and sinking fast. I paged Dr. McAuliffe and wasn't surprised that he was still in the hospital at that hour. He came right over to assist me, even though I wasn't part of his team and this patient wasn't his. What is most memorable to me, even after all these years, was the full hour he spent evaluating my patient. He asked detailed questions and listened carefully to the answers. He then performed the most thorough physical exam I've ever witnessed, probing every crevice of the patient's body, examining every fingernail, percussing and auscultating every organ. It was a medical tour de force. This was followed by a textbook-like note in the chart—single-spaced, red-pen script—methodically elaborating his evaluation, his reasoning, and his assessment.

Few physicians reach the pinnacle of Dr. McAuliffe in their examinations, but hopefully Jay received a reasonable initial evaluation. After that, it's a waiting game—waiting for the cultures to grow—but it's also a watching game, especially with neutropenic patients, who can decompensate faster than you can say MRSA.

If the culprit organism is sensitive to the antibiotics, the patient should start to improve in 24–48 hours. The fever should come down, and the blood pressure, pulse, breathing, and white-blood-cell count should begin to normalize. If not, it could be that different antibiotics are needed—that's the best-case scenario. The worst-case scenario is that the antibiotics were correct but sepsis has surged ahead on its own. Despite all our phenomenal medical advances, once you are behind the eight ball on sepsis, there's a good chance you'll never catch up.

During Jay's first 48 hours in the hospital, his clinical condition did not improve, and in fact it steadily worsened. Plotted out, his symptoms show that one organ system after another was being affected. His urine output decreased, a worrisome sign that his kidneys were failing. He had a swollen abdomen and right-upper-quadrant pain, suggesting that his liver was affected, possibly congested with fluid or (worse) harboring an abscess. His arms and legs swelled with fluid, suggesting that his vasculature was dilating and the vessels couldn't contain the fluid inside the vessel walls. Jay's hallucinations (his "altered mental status") indicated that his nervous system was being affected. This could have been delirium from the fever or a medication, but it could also have represented meningitis, encephalitis, or the spread of leukemia. His progressive difficulty breathing was a sign of pulmonary involvement. This could have represented fluid or blood clots in the lungs, pneumonia, the spread of cancer, or, as the hematology fellow initially speculated, ARDS. Mottling and discoloration of the skin suggested diminished blood supply to the skin.

And of course, Jay remained febrile throughout his time in the hospital—a strong indicator that the medical treatment was not gaining ground on the underlying infection. I wasn't present at Jay's bedside, and I well know that even serious changes in medical condition can creep up insidiously. Sometimes they are obvious only in retrospect. But even with those caveats, I was startled that no one on the medical team seemed to be reacting to Jay's relentless decline.

Dr. Peterson was a pulmonologist—the field from which critical-care specialists arise. The fellowship for pulmonologists (which they do after their medical residency) is, in fact, called "pulmonary/critical care." So if there's anyone in a hospital who should know when ICU-level care is required, it would be a pulmonologist.

Maybe Dr. Peterson didn't believe Jay's condition was serious. I recognize that it's dicey to render an opinion without being there and seeing exactly what he saw. Maybe the recent dose of morphine had calmed Jay's labored breathing just enough so that he appeared less sick at the moment that Dr. Peterson was at the bedside. But Jay was clearly gravely ill (he died five hours after the doctor's visit).

One thing that struck me about Dr. Peterson was that he seemed to wear only his "pulmonary" hat; the "critical-care" hat seemed to have been left in the staff locker room. His evaluation of Jay appeared to have focused solely on the lungs, and when he had satisfied himself that those two sacs of air were not the primary drivers of Jay's worsening condition, he exited the scene. It's true that after fellowship in pulmonary/critical care, some doctors focus their careers on the pulmonary aspect and some on the critical-care part (these latter docs are often called "intensivists" and spend their time running ICUs). It's likely that Dr. Peterson was of the pulmonary persuasion, which is perfectly fine, but you can't "unlearn" your training in critical care. I don't understand how Dr. Peterson could have filtered out the persistent fever, the abdominal pain, the dwindling urine output, the hallucinations, and the swollen limbs and made a beeline just toward the lungs with his stethoscope.

Which brings me to the conclusion that no one—not Dr. Peterson, not Dr. Mueller, not the nurses—seemed to be actually *looking* at the patient.

There's a famous clinical pearl passed on to medical students. The question asked is "How do you know when it's time to intubate a patient?" Medical students will typically reach for weighty data points for an answer—the oxygen saturation, the $CO_2$ level, the alveolar-arterial gradient. The answer from the wise senior resident is "none of the above." You make the decision based on *looking* at the patient. You should be able to tell from across the room when a patient needs to be intubated.

It's an oversimplified answer, perhaps, but it illustrates a key concept in medicine. It's easy to get inundated—and distracted—by the vast amounts of data spooling out from our medical machinery. Hundreds of data points are churned out every shift, and wading through them can be dizzying. Even experienced clinicians can miss the forest for the trees. Not to mention that our shortcut-loving brains tend to cherry-pick the data that reinforce what we want to believe.

The importance of stepping back and taking a good look at the patient in totality cannot be overstated, especially in confusing situations. Jay's case was complicated, no doubt: he had an uncommon and grave form of AML; he wasn't responding to standard antibiotics; he was exhibiting symptoms that didn't necessarily seem related. There was a bevy of medical people from different fields and different shifts involved, but it seemed as though each person on the team attended only to specific parts of Jay's case—the breathing, the knee, the skin color, the restlessness. No one seemed to look at the big picture or, frankly, at *him* as he labored under the weight of the implacable metabolic disintegration taking place within him.

It is true that the symptoms and ramifications of sepsis are varied and complex, and often tricky to sort out. The situation can be murky, especially initially, but with sepsis you don't have the luxury of waiting until things are clear—you have to act. The window of opportunity is not only slender but also ephemeral. Unlike some other diseases, sepsis does not wait until you've pinpointed exactly what's going on.

Which is precisely what happened with Jay. No one added up the signs and symptoms from each of Jay's organ systems. The nurses wrote off his symptoms as side effects of chemotherapy. The doctors didn't seem to find anything alarming enough to raise their own blood pressure. The overall clinical evaluation struck me as oddly lackluster, especially when you consider the location of the patient. Neutropenic fever and sepsis might be oddballs on an orthopedic ward, but this was a bone-marrow transplant unit. Every single patient on a BMTU, by definition, has an impaired immune system, from the disease or the treatment or both. One would expect a BMTU to be especially attuned to the risk of sepsis, in the way that a geriatrics ward is attuned to the risk of falls or a psychiatry ward is attuned to the risk of suicide.

So my conclusion about the clinical evaluation of Jay is that the recognition and diagnosis of sepsis seemed more sluggish than it should have been. But what about the treatment of his sepsis?

Antibiotics are a must for treating sepsis, but they aren't sufficient because the body's immune reaction is now running amok, unmoored from the underlying infection that triggered it. The main "treatment" for sepsis, therefore, is to keep the patient alive (what's demurely known as "supportive care"). You're trying to outfox and outlast the body's own self-damaging enterprise long enough for the antibiotics to do their thing. Keeping the patient alive, though, is a strenuous and fraught process.

The mainstay is aggressive hydration to support the collapsing circulatory system. As with burn patients like Glenn, aggressive hydration can easily backfire and cause fluid overload, because the blood vessels of septic patients are similarly over-dilated and inefficient at corralling fluid to where it needs to be. Finding the sweet spot between necessary, aggressive hydration and too much hydration requires deft medical management.

If fluid alone cannot maintain an adequate blood pressure, patients require pressors to artificially constrict the blood vessels to force blood supply to the critical organs. These medications, however, can strain the heart and cause arrhythmias. The over-constriction can paradoxically end up cutting off blood supply to the kidneys and other vital organs.

Septic patients are frequently in respiratory distress and often need intubation and mechanical ventilation. If the kidneys have been affected, emergency dialysis is sometimes needed. These supportive measures hopefully keep the patient alive until the antibiotics can work. But these treatments are immensely complicated and offer as many harms as they do benefits. As such, patients with severe sepsis are best managed in intensive care, which is why the best "treatment" for sepsis is early recognition and transfer to an ICU.

Would Jay have survived if he'd been transferred to the ICU earlier in the course of his sepsis? This is impossible to say. The mortality rate of sepsis ranges from 15% to 60% depending on how many organ systems have been affected. Jay's profound neutropenia and his particularly pernicious form of AML were severe handicaps. Earlier recognition of the sepsis with aggressive supportive care in the ICU would have offered him the best chance, but Jay might have died even with the most scrupulous medical treatment.

## NOT LISTENING TO THE SIGNIFICANT OTHERS

One of the perplexing aspects of this case is how little credence the staff gave to Tara's observations. Doctors see a patient once or twice a day on rounds for just a few minutes, and so they depend on nurses, who spend more time at the bedside. Nurses also have other patients to care for, and so often they rely on the patients—or family members and close friends—to let them know if anything is amiss.

Interactions between medical staff and family members run the gamut. Sometimes the interactions are smooth—good communication, mutual respect, plates of brownies—and the staff and family work together to enhance the patient's experience. But often it's less than ideal. Personalities, priorities, and bodies jab into each other in the cramped space of a stuffy hospital room. Resentment and disrespect can lead to downright hostility.

There's an additional element in the brew, however, when the family member is a medical professional. Some staff welcome relevant medical input, though others feel uncomfortable and judged. Medical family members can be useful additional sets of eyes on the patient, but they can sometimes give unwanted—or incorrect—medical advice.

Tara described very comfortable dealings with the staff during the induction chemotherapy and the initial outpatient visits: "Jay and I were treated with respect. We had nothing but positive interactions." But of course, things were going relatively well, medically, so there wasn't much to disagree on.

During the hospitalization for the neutropenic fever, though, the interactions became strained. It seemed that every time Tara tried to point out a worrisome sign, the medical staff reacted negatively. Did they think she was insinuating that their care was substandard? Did they view her as competition? Did they just not like her as a person?

It's impossible to know, obviously, if one hasn't witnessed the encounters. But it is disquieting that they seemed to ignore, even disparage, Tara's every concern. Many of her observations were objective—respiratory rate, heart rate, urine output (I's and O's). These hard data are a universal nursing vocabulary, and it seems strange that the staff nurses didn't respond to them, irrespective of their feelings toward Tara as a person. Perhaps it was an issue of nurse-on-nurse territoriality. Maybe it was a hierarchical issue of a high-power cancer center pooh-poohing a nurse from a community hospital. Or maybe they just wrote her off, on day one, as a "difficult" family member and simply tuned out anything she said.

Tara is the first to admit that she knew nothing about leukemia. "I was totally ignorant," she said. She checked out a textbook from the medical library hoping to get a good overview, but it turned out that the book was written for hematology specialists. ("I was out of my league," she recalled. "The first chapter kicked my ass!") Nevertheless, she soldiered on through the book, feeling that she owed it to Jay. It was that textbook that she was reading the first time she met Dr. Mueller, the Sunday morning after Jay was admitted with neutropenic fever.

"I saw her smirk when she read the title," Tara remembered. "It was unmistakable. Only over the years has it dawned on me that it must have rubbed her the wrong way. Dr. Mueller could have made light of it, or maybe offered me an easier read. Instead, she smirked." Tara quickly covered the book with her backpack and never brought it out again. But she noticed thereafter that the nurses were more curt with her, even though she was assisting them with much of the grunt work. "I was fetching Jay's water and changing his sheets and cleaning his BMs. I was helping them to keep track of his I's & O's, but something had changed, inexplicably."

Was Tara over-reading the situation? Was she being paranoid? Perhaps. In her view, they'd pegged her as "a frantic, overbearing, overanxious, bossy ER nurse from a podunk hospital in the middle of nowhere."

Again, I can't comment directly on this since I wasn't present. But I do know that doctors and nurses are expected—rightfully, in my opinion—to tolerate a range of responses from patients and their families. Illness is a stressor like almost no other. Panic, helplessness, worry, pain—these are everyday issues in a hospital, and they can turn even those with the most staid personalities into raving maniacs. And of course we know—or are supposed to know—that it is not, in fact, raving mania that we are seeing but fear and intense vulnerability. In some fields, you get to choose which clients you take on. In medicine, you don't. You take care of all your patients and their families, whether you like them or not. That's the job.

Maybe Tara was indeed frantic, overbearing, overanxious, and bossy. She may have been the most annoying, unpleasant family member on the entire ward. But all of that notwithstanding, her observations about Jay's progression to septic shock were largely correct. His cardiac arrest and death from sepsis sadly validated her clinical observations. The medical staff made an error—perhaps a fatal error—in not giving any credence to her words.

It's hard to imagine a more punishing way to be proved right.

## OVERCONFIDENCE IN CLINICAL ABILITIES

When Tara pressed Dr. Mueller about transferring Jay to the ICU, the hematologist responded, "Maybe in a smaller hospital he would be in the ICU, but not here." There's no doubt that a major cancer center has many capabilities that a community hospital can't possibly match. But as Mark Graber—the researcher on diagnostic error—had commented to me, "Overconfidence is an enormous problem, both personal and organizational."

One interesting study of overconfidence and medical error suggests that overconfidence is more of a problem in simple cases than in complex ones.[1] With difficult or unusual cases, doctors and nurses feel the chafe of their limitations and so tend to seek out guidance and additional knowledge. It's in situations that appear routine that overconfidence trips them up. The "metacognitive angst" caused by a complex case is absent, so staff members stop thinking and just perform rotely. I wonder if that's what might have happened in Jay's case. Dr. Mueller and the BMTU nurses kept viewing Jay's symptoms as a typical response to chemotherapy, and so perhaps they stopped thinking actively about what else might be going on.

I have to admit, though, that I was dumbstruck when Dr. Mueller said to Tara, "We don't electively intubate here at this hospital." It's one thing to say, "We don't do heart transplants here at this hospital" when a hospital doesn't possess such a facility. But it's quite another to say, "We don't do $X$," when $X$ is an available treatment in the realm of reasonability.

I could understand if Dr. Mueller had said, "We try to avoid elective intubation at this hospital," given that elective intubation certainly has harms. But such a statement would have been followed by "So here is what we do when a patient is having trouble breathing," with an elaboration of noninvasive respiratory methods such as BiPAP or a rundown of what respiratory therapists do.

The only circumstance in which I can imagine a doctor saying, "We don't electively intubate here at this hospital" is when a hospital doesn't own a ventilator. That might be the case in a rural hospital in a developing country, but it's a clear impossibility in a major hospital that performs high-risk procedures such as bone-marrow transplants. In any case, elective intubation is not a policy (as in, "We don't allow smoking here at this hospital") nor is it a medical practice that was once accepted but now disproven (as in, "We don't do blood-letting here at this hospital").

To say, "We don't electively intubate here at this hospital" would be like saying, "We don't do emergency C-sections here at this hospital." Nobody *wants* to deliver a baby under rushed conditions, but if the clinical situation warrants it, then you do it.

I have to at least consider the possibility that Dr. Mueller was completely clueless about sepsis. I find that a stretch because any hematology attending, even a junior one, has been through a residency's worth of clinical disasters and a fellowship's worth of cancer disasters. You don't have to preside over that many intubations—elective or emergent—to know this is something you do when you have to do it.

I can't say for sure that it was overconfidence in the abilities of the BMTU that led to Dr. Mueller's statement, but blunt fiat is a very limiting way of practicing medicine. Perhaps it was ego. Maybe having her treatment plan questioned—and implicitly doubted—by a nurse (or worse, a family member!) raised her hackles and she became defensive. We can never know exactly what prompted Dr. Mueller to write off elective intubation. But what we *can* see from the BMTU is that no one stepped up to take ownership of the situation, which to me is the defining error of Jay's case.

## LACK OF "OWNERSHIP" OF THE CLINICAL SITUATION

Caring for severely ill patients is never easy. And when the clinical condition is crumpling and the reasons aren't clear, it can be nearly as terrifying for the doctors and nurses as it is for the patient and family. There's a raw and ominous queasiness that creeps up on you when you sense the ground shifting under your patient and you're not exactly sure why. The permutations of pathology seem endless—infectious, inflammatory, metabolic, autoimmune, vascular, traumatic, toxic, neoplastic, congenital, iatrogenic, idiopathic—and the clinical progression can feel like it's spinning out of your control.

In the wake of confusion and decline it's tempting to plug the small holes, to chase the minutiae, to temporize until someone else's shift starts. This may net some gains on paper—the potassium level normalizes after supplementation; the fever is down after giving acetaminophen—but the underlying disease process hasn't been identified or controlled. This won't happen until someone takes ownership, both of the situation and of the patient.

Nowhere in the course of Jay's hospital stay did anyone seem to say, "This is my patient. I'm not going anywhere until I figure what's going on." This is not to imply that it's any one person's sole responsibility to understand and solve every clinical problem—that's not realistic, or even feasible. But it *is* the lead doctor's role to take ownership of the case, especially when things are not going well. This ownership comes in many forms. For starters, it involves clearing the deck—in your mind and, if necessary, in your schedule—to perform a head-to-toe evaluation at the patient's bedside. This should be followed by the equivalent amount of time sitting in the nurses' station thinking, analyzing the case from soup to nuts. You need to start from scratch and work your way methodically through the data and the clinical course to make sure you haven't missed anything. (Dr. McAuliffe was a master role model for this.)

Ownership might entail agitating the system to make things move faster—getting on the horn to CT and insisting on an abdominal scan stat. It might involve getting help, such as obtaining an infectious-disease consult, even in the middle of the night, because the patient remains febrile despite appropriate antibiotics. It might involve calling a colleague to get a second opinion, in this case maybe calling Dr. Everett, the outpatient hematologist who administered the chemotherapy and was familiar with Jay's medical intricacies. Ownership might involve acknowledging that you are in over your head and transferring the patient to the more appropriate setting.

Sometimes ownership is the physical act of planting your derriere at the bedside and not leaving until you know what's going on with your patient or your patient has stabilized or your patient has been moved to the appropriate clinical setting. But any way you slice it, ownership is taking full responsibility for your patient's care and not passing the buck. It doesn't mean you have to be a martyr who stays till 2 a.m. every night, nor does it mean you have to fly solo. But you do have to take on a leadership role and make sure the necessary things get done.

Whose job was it to take the leadership role in Jay's case? Twenty years ago there would have been just one primary doctor for both the inpatient and outpatient care. In that model, Dr. Everett—Jay's main hematologist for the AML—would have had the primary responsibility for Jay's care, whether it was during office visits, outpatient chemotherapy, or inpatient admissions. With the increasing complexity (and pace) of medical care, it has become unsustainable for a single physician do all the outpatient as well as the inpatient care, so many medical centers use the hospitalist model, under which full-time inpatient doctors ("hospitalists") assume the care when the patient is hospitalized.

But even this is an oversimplification. Patients are usually cared for by multiple consulting services who have commitments all over the hospital, and often at several different hospitals. Each of these consulting services might involve several levels of hierarchy—residents, fellows, attendings. The logistics alone make coordination of care a nightmare, but the real risk is diffusion of the sense of responsibility. It is very common, especially in complex cases, for each clinical service to "defer" to another service, leading to a serial punting of responsibility. No one takes charge.

In Jay's case, Dr. Mueller—the inpatient hematology attending on the BMTU—was the person who should have taken charge of this situation. As the senior doctor on the ward to which Jay was admitted, she had primary responsibility for his care. This is not to say that she was responsible for every iota of Jay's care or that every last fault in the case is on her shoulders, but it was her job to direct the care, coordinate the consultants, and make the final decisions. Most importantly, it was her job to take charge when the situation worsened. Instead, oddly, she seemed to pull back. This was the part that gave me the most pause.

In fairness, I did not have the opportunity to speak with Dr. Mueller, so I was not able to learn her perspective. In medicine—and in life—there are always nuances that don't meet the eye on initial gaze. Neutropenic fever is certainly well within the realm of what a hematologist deals with but perhaps there were clinical elements of the case that I am not aware of that drove her to different conclusions. Perhaps there was a personal antipathy toward Tara that got in the way. (We'd all like to think of medical staff as perfectly objective, but of course they are not.) Whatever it was, Dr. Mueller did not step up to the plate either in evaluating Jay's condition or in corralling the tests and treatments that he needed.

Dr. Peterson was a consultant, so he did not have primary responsibility for Jay's care. But even a consultant has to take ownership relevant to his or her part of the medical care. Again, I did not interview Dr. Peterson personally, so I cannot know what he was thinking, but it seemed to me that Dr. Peterson shirked his duty by limiting his consultation to the pulmonary aspect of the case and not including his full spectrum of critical-care knowledge.

The head nurse of a ward may not have the same legal responsibility as the attending physician, but that person is also expected to take ownership. If a patient is not getting the appropriate medical care, for whatever reason, it is the head nurse's job to stand up and insist that it happen. And if circumstances make this awkward or untenable, there is a strong chain of nursing leadership to turn to. Like her medical colleagues, Constance also seemed to pull back. I do not know how she was viewing matters in the moment, but from an outside perspective, it seems as though she did not take ownership of the situation or the patient. To her credit, though, she showed up at the meeting with Tara and expressed true remorse. She was the only member of the team who did so.

After Jay died, there was an autopsy. The pathologist found extensive colonies of MRSA spread throughout his body, along with evidence of sepsis-induced clots and bleeding, known as DIC (disseminated intravascular coagulation). The official cause of death listed on the death certificate was cardiopulmonary arrest secondary to sepsis.

While sepsis is challenging to identify and treat, it is a quantifiable subject that is eminently teachable. What is far harder to teach is responsibility and a sense of ownership. These concepts—"responsibility" and "ownership"—may be pasted into mission statements or hospital brochures, but they can't be taught in any meaningful way other than by example. When there are enough examples walking the halls of an institution, these values are infused into the culture and are absorbed by newcomers without any need for inspirational posters tacked onto the walls. They are among the rare things in medicine that we applaud for being contagious. Regrettably, lack of responsibility and ownership—as evidenced by Jay's experience—is also contagious.

Of all the emotions Tara experienced, the one that lingers undimmed—beyond grief—is disappointment. She was so tremendously disappointed in her fellow medical workers. For someone who took such pride in her work, this letdown was—and remains—profound.

"How was there no one to have helped Jay?" she continually wonders. "Not *one* nurse to say, 'Hey, this guy's circling the drain? Not *one* blessed CNA [certified nurse assistant] to actually count Jay's respirations for one minute rather than robotically write in the number 20? Not *one* oncologist to overrule the pulmonologist's recommendation of morphine rather than ICU transfer to address Jay's difficulty breathing? If I total all of the people who could have intervened on that day, I would include two physicians, two hematology fellows, one nurse manager, one case manager, two CNAs, and four nurses. My heart hurts to think about it."

But Tara also wonders if a single outspoken nurse could have actually made the difference. The entrenched power structure in medicine could easily have overridden that one clarion voice. Would that one lowly nurse have felt empowered to call a "rapid response" against the advice of the attending? And if a team had rushed to Jay's beside, might they have been turned away by a pulmonary specialist already at the bedside?

Jay's story caught my eye specifically because his wife was a nurse. Medical error devastates patients and families from any background, but I was intrigued to talk to someone on the patient side of things who was herself in the medical profession. One reason is that I wanted to equalize the knowledge balance. For many patients and families facing medical error, the knowledge imbalance can be an impenetrable hurdle. Having a family member who is fluent in neutropenia, hyperkalemia, BMTU, trisomy, and MRSA would eliminate that issue as a confounder.

But the second, and possibly more important, reason was that I wanted to explore the experience of medical error with someone who understands the twenty-plates-spinning-in-the-air reality of modern medicine. Nonmedical folks often have the impression that checking into a hospital is akin to stepping onto a Boeing 747. We peek into the cockpit and see a dizzying number of buttons and levers, but we allay our anxiety because we assume that every pilot knows every single one. All can be accounted for on a checklist. The number of buttons and levers in that cockpit may seem frightfully large, but it is a finite number.

Nonmedical folks assume that the hospital is a similarly circumscribed, smooth-running machine. Medical insiders, however, know that it's nothing like that. The number of variables—especially with critically ill patients—is vast, and the permutations and interactions of each are staggering. The variables don't just include every possible thing that can go wrong with every possible organ but also the sheer number of people involved in the care—nurses, doctors, therapists, fellows, attendings, CNAs, supervisors, technicians, medical students—and the rotations of each of the people in each of these roles, since every role must be covered twenty-four hours per day, seven days per week.

For those of us on the inside, working in a hospital does feel more akin to circus juggling. The potential for major error feels ever present. We are amazed that more plates *aren't* crashing to the ground. So I was interested to speak with someone who understood this dynamic.

Tara fit these two criteria. She was a clear-eyed realist who well understood the limitations of medicine and didn't harbor any false expectations. Her rapid-fire intellect made it easy to dig through the reams of clinical minutiae with her.

But there was a third aspect that arose that I hadn't really considered: the effect of the error on how that medical person would feel about her own profession and her own self as a member of that profession. I assumed there would be some frustration, even anger, but I hadn't given much thought to the depth and totality of these emotions. In retrospect, I should have, because I know how deep to the core the identity runs. For many doctors and nurses, medicine is not just a profession; it's a defining sense of self. In some other lines of work, you might hear, "I used to work in a bank, but now I'm in retail." But you never hear someone say, "I used to be a doctor" or "I was once a nurse." These professions define not what you *do* but who you *are*. A retired nurse never stops being a nurse, in her own eyes or in the eyes of the community. A retired doctor might say she's no longer in practice but would never say she's no longer a doctor. So I shouldn't have been surprised by the intense and utterly visceral nature of Tara's reaction.

"Betrayal" was the only word she could find to describe it. "The betrayal," she wrote to me, "runs as deep as I imagine people who have been victimized by molesting priests feel. I trusted in the healthcare system just as any devout Catholic trusts in the Catholic Church. I believed that the doctors making Jay's care plan were altruistic and adhered to their vow to 'First do no harm,' just as priests vow to be pious, chaste, and obedient. My healthcare profession was, to me, the way I felt closest to God. I had such faith in the work I was doing and in those who worked beside me.

"The nurses, in particular," Tara continued, "were supposed to be my professional sisters and brothers. We shared an understanding, so I thought, of the trenches of humanity during the most vulnerable time in patients' lives. We shared a belief—*didn't we?*—in delivering skilled nursing care coupled with compassion. We prided ourselves in the missed lunch breaks and UTI-inducing, bathroom-free, twelve-hour shifts, all in the name of patient care. Is there anything more honorable?

"The absolute spiritual betrayal of my fellow healthcare practitioners has so scarred me that it has taken years of sheer determination to undo. For nearly ten years afterward, my mirror reflected a rage-filled stranger."

CHAPTER SIXTEEN

# SO WHAT'S A PATIENT TO DO?

The anger and betrayal that Tara, Melissa, and Nancy suffered are a regretfully common experience for people who've lived through medical errors. And it's not surprising, since the medical system is supposed to be a refuge where you will be taken care of. Most people have a reasonable faith that things will go well. (Nurses routinely top the list of the most trusted professionals, followed by doctors and pharmacists.) So when things go wrong, it's a profound and painful breach.

Despite the ongoing and admirable efforts of the legions who are working to improve things, the reality is that healthcare is—and always will be—an imperfect system. Patients, unfortunately, have to stay alert and self-prescribe a healthy dose of skepticism. The popular press has moved nimbly to fill this need. Checklists and advice articles on how to stay safe in hospitals have sprung up everywhere. It's easy to get overwhelmed by all the tasks you as the patient are exhorted to do—make lists, check credentials, get second opinions, obtain copies of your X-rays, research medication interactions, figure out if your doctor receives industry payments, check on prior malpractice claims, keep your entire medical history on hand at all times, plus conduct a full-scale interrogation of anyone in scrubs who ventures within three feet of your epidermis. It's a tall order on your best days and downright punishing when you are preoccupied with being sick.

My take on the how-to-protect-yourself enterprise is less list-oriented and more perspective-oriented. If I had to pick one thing to focus on, it would be to recognize that healthcare—and I'll include here hospitals, doctors' offices, clinics, and emergency rooms—is a human endeavor. It's built by humans, researched by humans, and administered by humans. Too often there is the perception that the medical field is characterized entirely by scientific perfection. This is not to sell short the truly miraculous scientific advances that have, for example, transmogrified AIDS from a universal brutal killer into a manageable chronic disease in just a few years.

But there is a chasm of difference between the scientific certainty of medical progress as a whole (for an entire population) and the profound *uncertainty* of the medical experience for any given individual. This is the same frustrating gap we experience between the spectacular results of multimillion-dollar clinical trials and the impossibility of guaranteeing these eye-popping results for any given patient.

We all want zero medical errors—that's a no-brainer. But thinking with this all-or-none starkness does a disservice to the complexity of the situation as well as the reality. Every action we take involves a risk/benefit ratio. Crossing Third Avenue involves a risk/benefit ratio—we want the benefit of getting to the bagel store on the other side, but we take the risk that a driver might be inexperienced, or hung-over, or checking his phone. The benefit of getting that whole-wheat-everything bagel with lox and capers has to be balanced against the risk that we could get barreled down by two tons of beveled steel. The odds of getting run down are low, but the outcome of even a single instance is devastating. Thus every time we step off the curb, we have to consider the frequency of possible bad outcomes, the degree of badness of those outcomes, the necessity of getting across the street, and the impact of having to eat a stale hospital corn muffin for breakfast. And that's just one single decision.

The medical experience involves dozens of decisions, sometimes hundreds or thousands of decisions, trellised across the dizzying intricacies of the human body. The checklist model of the aviation industry does not sufficiently apply. Airplanes come in a finite number of models and within each model the planes are blessedly identical. Not so for humans, in whom the biological diversity of illness is further complicated by the even more varied layers of social factors that influence the disease process.

A more realistic way of approaching the medical experience is the concept of harm reduction. Can we rejigger things such that a patient will experience, say, five fewer errors during a hospital stay? Can we cut down medication mix-ups by 20%? Can we set up precautions so that the rate of falls in a nursing home will get cut in half? Such modest-sounding goals aren't what hospitals want to plaster on advertising billboards that line the nearby highways and airports. (For that, only cutting-edge, world-class, innovative, state-of-the-art phrasings need apply . . . and only if housed within Centers of Excellence, of course.)

Similarly, the modest goals of harm reduction also don't resonate with patients who rightly want zero errors in their medical care. Who'd want to go to a hospital that's striving to achieve 248 adverse events instead of 320? Who'd want to entrust their care to a place whose grand goal is to cut hospital-acquired infections by a lukewarm 22%?

But these admittedly lame-sounding incremental goals are the only ones that jibe with the reality of what can actually be achieved when trying to turn a gargantuan battleship like the healthcare system. If you demand zero medical errors, you will simply guarantee a gaming of the system and an over-reliance on meaningless buzzwords, a situation that is arguably even less safe for patients.

Harm-reduction strategies garnered big press with the AIDS and hepatitis C epidemics (and later with the opioid epidemic). They stoked controversy in the media because these medical crises involved populations, behaviors, and conditions that are easy fodder for moralizing—homosexuals, drug addicts, prostitutes, gay sex, multiple partners, needle-sharing, poverty. If everyone would just *behave*, the thinking went, these problems would no longer be problems. However, for the people in the trenches—both patients and healthcare workers—it was abundantly clear that such lofty admonitions weren't making much of a dent. Patients were dying in droves, and putting a dent in the decimation was urgently needed, by whatever means would work. Distributing free condoms and providing clean needles for intravenous drug users were practical ways to bring down the death rate in the immediate term, allowing medical research to take the painstaking time needed to develop better treatments.

These harm-reduction strategies irritated many policymakers because they seemed to accept and even "encourage" unacceptable behaviors. But they actually saved lives. Not all lives, of course, but fewer patients contracted HIV and hepatitis C. Fewer patients died. The harm-reduction strategies didn't solve everything but they did reduce the burden of suffering that patients experienced. The same can be said for distributing naloxone kits to reverse opioid overdose, and offering methadone and buprenorphine for patients with opioid addiction. They save lives and buy time.

These strategies don't sugarcoat the very real dangers of drug use and unprotected sex. Rather, they evince a practical recognition that these dangerous things do exist, but that we can nevertheless work to minimize the harm they cause.

Similarly, medical error is a reality in medical care that won't easily or quickly—or likely ever—be fully eradicated. But the prevalence and severity of error can be minimized with a harm-reduction approach (while medical research works to develop systemic solutions).

So what can you do as a patient to minimize harm? For starters, it's important to know your own medical history. This may seem like an obvious point, but I'm always surprised by how many patients have trouble with this. It's a good idea to make a one-page list that has your basic diagnoses, your current medications and the dosages, what surgeries you've had, and what you are allergic to.

Resist the urge to create a forty-page, single-spaced, cross-referenced treatise that lists every cold you've had, your teenage acne, your stubbed toes, and the fact that garlic powder gives you the hiccups. Keep it simple, clear, and relevant. (An exception can be made if you've had a complex treatment such as chemotherapy or a heart transplant. For that, you can keep a separate sheet that includes the nitty-gritty details.)

Having a basic info sheet on hand for any medical encounter can help prevent basic errors like prescribing something you are allergic to or that is contraindicated based on one of your conditions.

Medications change frequently, so it is wise to compare your medication list to your doctor's list at every visit. The most practical way to do this is to sweep your pill bottles into a bag and bring it with you. I find this to be the most helpful method, because sometimes there are medications prescribed by other doctors that I wouldn't otherwise know about. Or the dosage of a medication was changed at an urgent-care visit. If you take supplements, herbal medications, or over-the-counter meds, throw them in their own bag and bring it along too.

When it comes to minimizing diagnostic error, the focus should be on the conversation. The conversation between the patient and the medical team is the single most critical diagnostic tool, so you want to make sure it does not get short shrift. If your doctor has not unglued her eyes from the computer screen for the entire visit and is robotically filling in check boxes, you are well within your constitutional rights to politely point that out. You could say something like, "I know that you have to write all this down in the computer, but if you could give me one minute of your full attention, I'll tell you the important stuff as concisely as possible." You want to be sure you are having a thorough, engaged conversation with your doctor so that your symptoms can be adequately explored.

And when your doctor says, "I think you have X," you should ask, "What makes you think so?" This will help you understand how convinced (or not) your doctor is by the data. Then ask, "Is there anything else that it could be?" This will provide insight into the doctor's differential diagnosis and clinical reasoning. If you want to press further, you could ask, "Is there anything we can't afford to miss?" If your doctor turns out to be someone who snaps to a quick diagnosis, these simple questions will force her to engage in the reasoning process she should have done all along.

Infection is one area where there is a practical strategy for prevention. Make sure you witness every medical person wash their hands before they touch you. Make a joke if you must, be self-deprecating, neurotic, or forceful if you need to be, channel your inner Ignaz Semmelweis if you can, but do whatever it takes to keep germ-laden hands off you until they've been washed with soap or thoroughly rubbed with a waterless disinfectant. (If your doctor or nurse acts affronted, maybe try asking them in which of Semmelweis's two obstetric clinics would *they* want to get their medical care?)

For hospitalized patients (and for anyone undergoing extensive outpatient treatment such as chemotherapy), perhaps the most critical safety feature is the presence of another person. It is simply too much to ask a person who is acutely ill or receiving bulldozer-level medical treatments to keep track of the intricacies of what is going on. If you are puking your guts out or bone-rattling from a 104 degree fever, you have enough on your plate. You've earned your dispensation to focus on the immediacy and awfulness of being sick.

The second person has to be your eyes and ears. That person should keep a notebook at the bedside and write down—and ask about—every single thing that transpires. What is the diagnosis? What is this medication for (and how do you spell it)? What side effects should you look out for? What are today's blood test results? Who is this 37th person in a white coat? Why is the patient getting a CT scan? (And how good is a CT scan for this issue?) When should we expect a response to the treatment?

It can be hard to speak up. And even when you do—as Tara experienced— it can be even harder to effect change. Still, family members and friends are essential for keeping tabs. The very act of having the medical team clarify each step—and, crucially, the thought process behind each step—is a good check on common medical errors. The staff might give you a Tony Award for being the most annoying family member on the ward, but that's okay. (You can always drop off a box of cookies to soothe ruffled egos.) Asking questions and writing down the details provides a paper trail during a confusing journey. And should something go wrong, it's an invaluable tool for reconstructing the timeline.

Midway through writing this book, a Friday-night stomachache on the part of my teenage daughter landed us in the ER. As a rule, I do not overreact to the aches and pains of everyday life. Fevers, colds, coughs, and sprained ankles do not get my pulse up. My children know that "if you're not bleeding out or having cardiac arrest," their mother isn't putting down the *New York Times*, except perhaps to recount stories of her patients who are *actually* sick, occasionally annotated with unrequested teaching points like how the liver has two different blood supplies—*isn't that so cool?* If they want medical sympathy, they know they need to go to their computer-programmer father.

But this time I became suspicious of her inability to find a comfortable position and so pulled out my stethoscope. When I heard complete silence instead of gurgling bowel sounds, I grabbed our coats and shuttled us straight to the ER. My correct diagnosis of appendicitis evidently redeemed me as a doctor in my daughter's eyes, though she was mortified that I chatted it up with the various colleagues who crossed our path. (Ahem, appendicitis does *not* preclude basic rules of civility.)

Surgery was scheduled for the next morning, and she spent the night in a hospital room receiving IV fluids and pain medications. I found that I was unable to sleep, despite my fatigue. It surely didn't help that I was reviewing journal articles about medical error for this book during my daughter's interludes of fitful sleep. Whenever anyone entered the room, I jumped up to scrutinize who they were and why they were there.

When the pediatric resident arrived at 3 a.m. to take my daughter's history—after she'd told her story to (and been examined by) the triage nurse, the ER resident, the ER attending, the surgery resident, the surgery chief, and then the surgery attending—I put my foot down. I forbade the resident from waking her up for what seemed like the seventeenth time.

"But we have to," the resident said.

As a doctor, I knew that this was the standard protocol. But as a parent I was incensed, though I knew that anger wasn't a practical strategy for getting anything accomplished. Better to approach this as a teaching moment. "What do you think you might find," I asked, as Socratically as one can be at that hour of the night, "that would *change* your diagnosis or management?" The resident hesitated. I took the opportunity to plow forward with a clinical-reasoning lesson. I was a faculty member of her institution, after all. "She's on pain meds now, so you won't find any tenderness on physical exam. The ultrasound has already shown an inflamed appendix, and her white count is elevated. If there is something on history or physical that would suggest that surgery is *not* indicated, by all means proceed."

The resident eyed me warily, fingering her stethoscope while I felt myself transmogrifying from didactic doctor to pissed-off parent. "But if you are going to wake her up, jab on her belly, and then come to the grand conclusion that she has appendicitis and needs surgery, forget about it," I snapped. "Let the poor kid sleep."

Another long pause. I could sense that the resident was calculating the risk/benefit ratio of pressing her case with an ornery, sleep-deprived parent. "You can write 'parent refuses H&P' in the chart," I offered helpfully. The resident ultimately backed off, and I flopped back into my chair to read yet another cheery article about medical disasters.

At one point, the surgery team offered the option of giving *just* IV antibiotics instead of doing surgery. The idea was that some patients could be spared an operation. With antibiotics alone, they said, there was a roughly 50% chance of appendicitis recurring at some later date. Which meant that for half the patients, surgery could be avoided altogether. This sounded promising—who wouldn't want to avoid surgery if possible?—but the team said we had to decide right now so they could know whether to book the OR for the morning.

I'm not a surgeon and I'm not a pediatrician, so this is not my area of expertise. I asked the surgery resident whether this recommendation was based on some preliminary study of fifteen patients, or had there been a solid trial with hundreds of patients followed for ten years? The resident heaved a sigh, and I could tell he wasn't thrilling to the idea of dissecting the data in the middle of the night with an annoying parent/attending when he surely had a scut list a mile long.

But we needed to know not just that there were two alternatives available but how the alternatives stacked up against each other. I wasn't going to make a half-baked decision just because the team was time-pressed to get the OR schedule ready.

With cajoling and a few strategic Internet searches, we pulled up some of the studies. The data for antibiotics were a bit preliminary but encouraging, especially for someone who might be frightened of surgery. Now I should tell you that my daughter is not a fan of needles of any stripe. Getting a flu shot reduces her to a sobbing mess who has to huddle in my lap—quite literally— for the vaccination, even though she's a head taller and a stone heavier than me. I was sure she'd jump at the chance to avoid surgery, with its attendant scalpels and other sharp-edged paraphernalia.

It turned out that she had an utterly different take on it. The experience of being in the ER and getting IVs was so miserable that she never *ever* wanted to repeat it. The definitiveness of surgery was much more appealing to her than the possibility—however small—of going through all of this again at some time in the future. Besides, she'd already suffered the pain of getting the initial IV in the ER, and she calculated that it could be used all the way through the next day. Undergoing general anesthesia and surgery seemed to her like a very reasonable way of avoiding having an IV at a future date!

All in all, the decision to choose the standard treatment of surgery took several hours, not several minutes. We did not win any kudos for being the easiest-to-manage patients, but I felt we'd done the right thing by forcing the team to articulate the relative strengths of the treatment options and also to factor in the patient's values and preferences, even if they were somewhat inflected with teenage myopia.

The hospitalization proceeded smoothly, though there was an excruciating moment in the OR the next morning when my daughter was getting onto the table. She hadn't been expecting quite so many masked and gowned bodies looming over her, and the oxygen mask descending upon her probably felt smothering. She suddenly panicked and began fighting off the medical team, screaming my name and begging me to help her. I was already being led out of the room, but my parental instinct was to rush over and save her. Instead I had to give permission for—and then witness—the staff wrestle my terrified child back onto the table and forcibly corral the mask over her face. I knew the anesthetic would kick in within seconds, and that she'd likely have little recollection of this, and that going forward with surgery was the right thing to do for her. But still, it was parental agony.

And then there was the lighter moment, post-op, when she was coming out of anesthesia. I asked her if she'd like some Toradol, the pain medication that the nurse was offering. My daughter's speech was still slurred, but my words had clearly penetrated her consciousness. "Tortellini?" she mumbled, and there was a faint but noticeable lift in her voice. "Are we having tortellini?"

In the end, it was a success. That dangly tail of residual colon was successfully snipped out, and we were home before bedtime that night. I was impressed, yet again, by the marvels of modern medicine, knowing full well that had this taken place a century earlier I might have been digging a grave for my child that evening instead of digging through the freezer to see if we had any tortellini.

I also marveled, yet again, at just how many moving parts exist in a hospital. As a physician who is part of this enterprise, I'm stunningly proud of the breadth of medical care our hospital can provide—handling everything from gallstones and premature infants to limb reattachments and acute psychosis. But during our stay as patients, every one of these wonderful moving parts looked to me like a medical error waiting to happen. The sheer number of people who traipsed in and out of my daughter's room was staggering, and all I could think about was how many different microbial colonies they were pummeling into the mix, each with its own scurrilous array of infectious possibilities.

To the untrained eye, it's virtually impossible to tell who is who; everyone from the housekeeper to the surgeon wears some version of scrubs. Even to the trained eye it's challenging. ID cards dangle amid keys and pens, and they are impossible to read even if it isn't the middle of the night in a darkened room and your glasses are lost in the muddle of bedside tissues, ice chips, and ginger ale. And this was just a case of uncomplicated appendicitis. When you are *really* sick, it can feel like the entire population of a midsize city is trekking to your bedside, usually at the most inopportune moments possible.

I wasn't a complete ogre to everyone, of course. (Well, maybe a little.) I just wanted a clear justification for each procedure. And it had to carry more weight than "This is what we do." I'm sure I slowed down the workflow and ruffled more than a few feathers. But addressing family members' worry about medical error is part of the job—even if the family member isn't a physician, and isn't on the faculty of the institution, and doesn't coincidentally happen to be writing a book about medical error while sitting at the bedside. It is—or should be—standard-of-care for every patient.

Of course, the burden should not have to be on the patient or family for ensuring good and safe medical care. That is the job of the healthcare system. But as we well know, the system has not quite achieved pristine perfection, so it behooves patients and families to stay engaged in the details as much as they can. You don't necessarily need to be in full vulture mode, as I was, but you do need to be persistent and not care if the staff think you are annoying.

No one likes to be the squeaky wheel, especially in a system that exudes the not-so-subtle message that everything will run smoother with docile, compliant patients. I can understand why Tara felt defeated and chose, at times, to keep her thoughts to herself. It's not easy to be a gadfly, even when someone's life depends on it. My advice is to be polite but persistent. It can help to acknowledge that everyone is working hard and trying to do the right thing—offer appreciation for the things that are going well—but then plow forward with your questions and concerns.

For the patient who *doesn't* have a family member or trusted friend willing or able to sit at the bedside, it's a terrible conundrum. What do you do if you are alone? This is a very real and very difficult circumstance. My advice is to keep your own notebook, to the best of your ability. Jot down as much as you are capable of. At the very least, ask what each medication is and why you are getting it. The nurse can write it down for you or print out a list. And if you are too nauseated or too sleepy or too feverish to engage in discussion, don't rack yourself with guilt because you are not cross-examining every staff member. Get the rest you need. Before you doze off, though, use some of the leftover surgical tape to affix a sign across your chest that says "Wash your hands!"

---

What happens, though, if something does go wrong? What should you do if you think an error or an adverse event has occurred? Personally, I believe in direct communication. I would ask your doctor or nurse to explain what happened. It's human nature, however, to become defensive when something goes wrong, so you will likely get the best results if you resist the prosecutorial urge. Be low-key and constructive. Convey that your goal is to simply understand the facts of what transpired.

If you don't get satisfactory answers, ask to speak to a supervisor. There's always a chain of command that you can work your way up. (Keep track in your notebook of whom you've spoken to, when you reached out, and whether you heard back.) Most healthcare organizations have a patient advocate on staff. This is someone you can contact at any point in your search for information—or at any point in your medical care. Patient advocates are there for you, so you should feel completely comfortable calling on them. Your health insurance company may also have an advocate on staff, as might your employer or union. Take liberal advantage of these.

The other entity to be aware of is the risk management office. This is the team that is ultimately responsible for anything that goes wrong in a hospital. In the ideal world, risk managers are advocating wholeheartedly for patients, but their job is to look out for the hospital's best interests. Often these interests align, but you can imagine scenarios in which they don't, so keep that in mind.

Always request copies of your medical records. By law, you own the information in the chart, since it is all about you. It can sometimes be laborious to obtain your chart—forms to fill out, copying fees to pay—but don't let anyone tell you that you can't access the information. It is yours.

Outside the medical system itself, there are other resources. If your issue is primarily with an institution rather than an individual doctor, you can file a complaint with the Joint Commission, the major accrediting body in the United States. The Joint Commission is verbally referred to as "Jay-Co," based on the former, unpronounceable acronym JCAHO (Joint Commission on Accreditation of Healthcare Organizations). The triennial inspections by this body inspire fear, headaches, mountains of paperwork, and frenzied repainting of walls in nearly equal amounts. JCAHO eventually made a formal name change so as to be officially known as the "Joint Commission." This did nothing to decrease the dread of their visits, but did inspire a wave of hospital-corridor grumblings about how much marijuana was needed to deal with the stress of the inspections.

The Joint Commission is not a government organization but rather a private company charged with regulating hospitals, laboratories, nursing homes, clinics, homecare services, and mental health centers. If you have experienced an adverse event that is related to how one of these institutions runs, you can file a complaint with the Joint Commission. You can also contact your local board of health, as Melissa and Nancy did regarding Glenn's care.

If your error relates to an individual doctor, nurse, or other healthcare worker, you can file a complaint with the state board for each of these professions. Doctors or nurses found to be have been negligent can be disciplined or—in extreme cases—have their licenses revoked.

Other resources can be found on the website of the National Patient Safety Foundation. As well, there are many local patient-advocacy organizations, such as the one that Peter Mullenix became involved with.

What if none of these help? Should you get a lawyer? Although television dramas make it seem easy, stepping into the legal system is not for the faint of heart. If you are not fortunate enough to live in Scandinavia, you must prepare for a years-long slog. Keep in mind the sobering fact that the vast majority of "adverse events" will not be appropriate for litigation. You must be able to prove that your care was substandard *and* that the substandard care was the cause of the harm you experienced. Moreover, the harm has to be significant enough to generate a substantial financial need (such as severe disability, loss of life, or major medical bills). Otherwise the compensation won't cover the cost of litigating the case. The malpractice route will help only a tiny sliver of patients.

As Tara, Melissa, and Nancy learned, dealing with a medical error is never easy. Although the steps on paper seem clear, the reality is slow, painful, and rarely gratifying. And even if you receive acknowledgement, apology, and sometimes financial remuneration, the errors themselves can't be undone. The physical and emotional damage, sadly, are often permanent. This is something that we in the medical profession need to take responsibility for. We can't escape the reality that our ministrations can sometimes cause harm. It's our duty to do everything to minimize and avoid harm, but when things go wrong, we owe our patients a full-throated reckoning.

# CHAPTER SEVENTEEN

# GETTING IT RIGHT

Much of this book has focused on two singularly tragic cases. Jay and Glenn experienced some of the harshest iterations of our modern healthcare system. I chose these cases to highlight because of the many lessons they offer (and of course because of the remarkable generosity of their families).

But in some ways, Jay's and Glenn's cases are atypical of medical error. For one, they represent the catastrophic end of the medical-error spectrum, whereas most medical errors—though equally important to tackle—do not cause such harm. The other way in which their cases are less typical is the degree of inadequate medical care. In fairness, I was not able to interview the medical staff in these two cases, nor was I privy to the full details of the medical records or the negotiated settlements. But from what I could gather as an outsider (and from reviewing these cases with experts), some aspects of the recognition and treatment of these two severe conditions—sepsis and burns—fell glaringly short. I can't use the legal term "negligence"—again, I don't have all sides of the stories—but the medical care in both cases seemed wanting.

These cases of flagrant mismanagement and the seemingly uncaring attitude of medical staff are what make headlines and are thus what most people think of when they imagine medical error. But in reality, most errors are made by conscientious and competent staff who care deeply about their patients. These doctors and nurses are not perfect—that's for sure—and many are not as good as they could be or should be. But when they make an error or somehow harm their patient, most are torn to shreds with remorse.

The thing that *is* typical about Jay's and Glenn's cases is that medical error is rarely one thing only. A bad outcome is most often the result of multiple errors snowballing on top of each other. And what these cases most exemplify, in my opinion, is that tragic outcomes usually result from a combination of specific checklist-able items (like when to remove a catheter or when to transfer to a burn center) and those less tangible qualities, such as clinical reasoning, intellectual humility, effective communication, and a sense of ownership.

As we try to make the medical system safer for patients, we have to consider both aspects. The less tangible qualities are the hardest to imbue. They can only be created by boots on the ground, by people who exemplify these traits, teach these skills, and demand comparable behavior from their colleagues. The concrete items are logistically easier to approach, and that's where most healthcare organizations focus their efforts. However, it's not possible to bombard the staff with 3,471 checklists—though some hospitals certainly try. We need to rejigger the system to make it less possible for people to commit errors.

Human-factors engineering is the budding field that examines how people interact with the tools and technologies around them, and uses logical design to make things intrinsically safer. A simple example is the food processor that sits on nearly every kitchen countertop. The whirring blades could easily sever fingertips if a person reached in for a taste while, say, pulverizing cauliflower. Using the principles of human-factors engineering, the designers created a system in which the motor is unable to start unless the cover is locked into place. So if your brain falls under a cruciferous swoon, unable to control its urges to snag some beguiling florets in *flagrante delicto*, the machine will outsmart you and click off as soon as you open it.

I discussed a comparable example earlier in the book, in which anesthesiologists can no longer mix up nitrogen and oxygen in the operating room because the tubing and connectors are no longer interchangeable. The healthcare system is riddled with opportunities like this, where the system could be revamped to help humans make fewer errors. Often, however, they come to light only after a tragedy.

Heparin is potent blood thinner that is used to treat blood clots. In a far more diluted form, heparin is also used to flush catheters and IVs in order to prevent the tubes from clogging. In 2006, six premature infants in Indiana had their catheters accidentally flushed with the more concentrated heparin. Three of them died.

In examining the error, hospitals realized that the diluted and concentrated heparin came in identically sized vials, and that you had to squint at the label to distinguish them. The manufacturer issued a safety alert and changed the labels so they would be easier to tell apart. Unfortunately, not all hospitals had removed the old vials, and a year later three more infants in California accidentally received the concentrated dose. Luckily, none died, but it pointed out that human-factors engineering has to be thought out carefully.[1]

Hospitals had to take more drastic steps, like physically removing the vials of concentrated heparin from the general wards. They also switched to prefilled syringes that were of different sizes entirely.

Other ways that human-factors engineering can be used to reduce medical error include the physical architecture of hospitals and clinics. We know that handwashing is the most critical technology for infection control, but sinks are often inconveniently located, based more on the plumbing geography than anything else. Hospitals could be proactively designed to allow sinks to be closer to patients, where doctors and nurses are more likely to use them. However, if the sinks are poorly designed, they themselves can become vectors for spreading infections. Sinks that gush straight into the not-so-clean drains, for example, can cause splashback, and this has been implicated in outbreaks of infection in several hospitals.

There's more geographic flexibility with alcohol-based hand sanitizers. They can be placed just about anywhere, but it's amazing how often they manage to be in inconvenient locations. The one in my exam room, for instance, forces me to turn my back to the patient every time I wash my hands. Besides forcing me to be rude to my patients, it deprives the patients of their ability to accurately monitor the safety situation. If we want patients to be empowered to point out things like doctors forgetting to wash hands, they need to be able to see it. And of course, alcohol-based sanitizers are not a complete substitute for handwashing. While they inactivate microorganisms, they don't necessarily kill them. Notably, they don't work for C. diff, the organism responsible for much of hospital-acquired diarrhea. Additionally, as anyone who uses sanitizers eighty-five times per day can tell you, their desiccating power is prodigious, and most of us walk around with appendages that resemble prunes imported from the Kalahari.

Human-factors engineering for infection control can strategize beyond facilitating handwashing and look for ways to decrease the squatting rights of hospital microbes. Simple things such as shortening the sleeves on lab coats and outlawing neckties could keep dangly material from sweeping bacteria from patient to patient. Bed rails—perhaps the prime dalliance site for hands and bacteria—could be made of antimicrobial materials such as copper. The privacy curtains that surround beds and exam tables—as well as lab coats and scrubs—could be made of material that is less hospitable to microorganisms. Though handwashing remains the primary way to prevent spread of infection, these types of designs can act as a check on cognitively overloaded humans who occasionally forget to wash their hands.

An idea that shows promise for decreasing medication error is the creation of what are known as medication safe zones in pharmacies and nursing stations. These safe zones would include revolutionary features such as bright lighting and magnifying glasses to read fine print. They would also organize medications in cognitively logical ways. Rather than just alphabetize everything, for example, the system could be set up so that commonly used medications are easier to access, or so that everything needed for an IV setup is located together.

Most importantly, though, these safe zones acknowledge the need for mental focus. In a typical nursing station, you can hardly maintain a train of thought to successfully scratch your left ear, given the blizzard of phones ringing, alarms blaring, staff crisscrossing, housekeepers mopping, patients requesting ginger ale, wandering visitors looking for their loved ones, clueless medical students who can't work the electronic thermometer, post-call surgery residents hoping to score leftover donuts, a transporter waiting impatiently to bring Mr. Atkins to radiology, and then the nursing supervisor swooping in to remind everyone to be shipshape because of the upcoming Joint Commission inspection. Oh, and the EMR will be down for the next few hours because of a new roll-out, for which there will be a required in-service instruction session, but there aren't enough staff to cover, so every third nurse will be floated to a different unit. Oh, and the staff restroom is out of order again, so you'll have to use one on a different floor; please stagger your bathroom breaks accordingly.

While I exaggerate perhaps a touch, this is not so far off from the reality of a typical nursing station in a busy hospital ward. It would be challenging to invent an environment *less* conducive to the dogged thoroughness that is required to get every medication right every time for every patient, which is, of course, what is expected. The goal of medication safe zones, therefore, is to create secluded, quiet places that are free from distractions. A nursing station could be designed with a recessed room that physically barricades the nurse from the bedlam of the ward. Nurses preparing medications might even wear snazzy safety vests of fluorescent orange, so that everyone else knows to back off and shut up.

When it comes to diagnostic error—perhaps the toughest nut to crack—I think about the need for similar distraction-free zones in order to think critically about a patient's diagnosis. The crush of EMR documentation, however, snuffs out any possible semblance of contemplation. Our current model of indentured EMR servitude saps the vigor of even the most committed clinician. If we want medical staff to apply Graber and Singh's cognitive discipline about creating a differential diagnosis, questioning data that don't fit, examining our thought processes for bias, doubling back to ensure we didn't miss anything crucial—well, our neurons will need some time and space to strut their stuff. Something will have to give. Either we decide that there needs to be more time in a visit (which is ultimately a financial decision) or we have to radically scale back the documentation demands to allow clinicians time to actually think.

With all the talk of how the digital revolution will rescue healthcare, and how creative disruption will bulldoze us into a technology-infused nirvana, I look at the idea of medication safety zones and find it mildly ironic that one of the biggest "innovations" in patient safety is the concept of peace and quiet. But there you have it: one of the key ways to decrease medical errors is to allow nurses and doctors time and space to think. Uninterrupted. (And while we're at it, such peace and quiet would be highly salutary for patients, who can hardly get two consecutive winks of sleep in the hospital on account of all of our sophisticated technology.)

---

Improving patient safety ultimately requires a shift in the culture. Our traditional definition of medical error is things that go palpably wrong, like operating on the wrong side of the body or giving the wrong medication. But many things that we once took for granted as "regrettable but expected" side effects of medical treatment—like catheter-associated infections and pressure ulcers—are now viewed as preventable.

In the traditional fee-for-service system, insurance companies would pay for whatever medical care was delivered. Increasingly, though, insurers don't want to pay for things that shouldn't have happened. In 2008, Medicare initiated a "nonpayment program" in which it declined to reimburse hospitals for conditions it viewed as preventable. These hospital-acquired conditions included urinary infections, bloodstream infections, falls, blood clots, transfusion of incorrect blood type, and uncontrolled blood glucose levels. In a before-and-after analysis of more than 800,000 patients in 159 hospitals, the years following the implementation of this nonpayment program showed a distinct decline in these conditions, especially infections.[2]

There is no doubt that squeezing hospitals in the pocketbook gets them to focus harder on these preventable harms. One hopes that hospitals achieve these improvements by investing in the appropriate resources—adequate nurse staffing, an EMR that doesn't lobotomize its users—but of course there's always the human instinct to game the system. When Medicare began penalizing hospitals when too many patients were readmitted quickly (suggesting inadequate treatment), hospitals developed "observation units" where read-mitted patients could stay for up to 23 hours. These observations units were considered "outpatient," so, technically, patients were not actually admitted to the hospital (even if they were lying in hospital beds, wearing hospital gowns, and eating the same unpalatable hospital food). While observation units have many legitimate purposes, there is no doubt that some hospitals use them to artificially tamp down their readmission numbers and avoid the fines.

Another aspect of the necessary culture shift is in the vantage point we use to fix medical error. Most often, we approach errors with hindsight—something bad happens, and we address it after the fact. This is a laborious process, as investigations can take months, and implementing changes can take even longer. Moreover, this process usually relies on someone volun-tarily reporting the error. Even if a medical professional is able to overcome the discomfort of owning up to an error, the reporting systems can be so arduous to use—*please create a temporary password with at least three Cyrillic numerals, two capitalized Latin declensions, plus a fungal species of your choice*—that even the best Samaritans are defeated. Most experts estimate that less than 10% of adverse events or errors ever come to light, though admittedly this is impossible to measure.

What if we could set up a system that could detect errors automatically? Even better, what if the system could detect errors in real time? Put another way, if we are all going to be manacled to the EMR anyway, we may as well harness its power and use it to catch errors as they are happening. Infection-control teams have been doing a version of this for years. Microbiology labs track culture results to uncover clusterings that suggest incipient infection outbreaks. However, there are only a finite number of variables that humans can track.

With the EMR, it's possible to track all patients with infection—every single place in the hospital they've been, every staff member they've been in contact with, every medication they've taken, who their roommates were, ex-actly when their samples turned positive, what diet they were prescribed—and compare all of these data to patients who did not get infected to figure out which factors are spreading infections.

One hospital used this to track an outbreak of the energetically conta-gious C. diff bacteria, the bug mentioned earlier that isn't killed by hand sanitizers. C. diff (*Clostridium difficile*) infection provokes massive diar-rhea and can be deadly. The bacteria sheathe themselves in cleanser-resistant spores, which hop happily from hands to beds to sheets to instruments to sinks as patients shuttle through the various departments of the hospital, sending epidemiologists and housekeepers on ceaseless chases with gallons of bleach. (The name "difficile" was given because culturing it in the lab was so difficult, back when the bacillus was first identified in 1935. The appellation remains apt because it's so damn difficult to eradicate.)

In this hospital, the voluminous EMR churned data for more than 86,000 admissions, including more than 400,000 patient-location changes.[3] A sophisticated analysis was able to pinpoint the source of the outbreak to a single CT scanner located in the emergency room. Digging deeper, the team uncovered the reason for the outbreak: the radiology department had updated its protocol for cleaning CT machines, but apparently the news hadn't reached the ER. The ER radiology suite was still employing the older technique, which was clearly no match for the tenacious C. diff.

The glut of data generated by EMRs thus offers the tantalizing possibility of picking up errors as they are happening. The Global Trigger Tool, developed by the Institute for Healthcare Improvement, is one such algorithm that uses the EMR to identify potential trouble spots. It's important to note that these are "potential" trouble spots and must be investigated to determine if something untoward is actually occurring. For example, use of diphenhydramine (Benadryl) is considered a trigger because it's given in response to allergic reactions and anaphylaxis. However, it's also given as a sleep aid or if a patient suffers from seasonal allergies. Whenever diphenhydramine is used, a red flag would snap to attention in the EMR, but a human being would have to check to see whether the patient was having an allergic reaction to her medications or whether a visitor was wearing a cardigan knitted from cat hair.

Triggers, then, aren't automatic indicators of errors or adverse events, but they suggest that there is a good possibility and thus should be investigated in real time. Deployment of the code team or a rapid response team is a trigger, as is unplanned dialysis. Other triggers include a patient returning to the emergency room within 48 hours, or returning to the operating room a second time, or being readmitted to the hospital within 30 days. All of these are clues that something amiss might be happening.

Triggers include certain lab values—very low or very high blood sugar, elevated lactate (suggesting sepsis), or rapid decline of kidney function or blood counts. Other triggers are blood clots noted on CT scans or ultrasounds, administration of vitamin K (an antidote for the blood thinner warfarin), patient falls, the need for physical restraints, and the development of pressure ulcers.

In hospitals that have piloted the Global Trigger Tool, about ten times as many "safety events" are uncovered compared with hospitals that use the standard voluntary reporting method.[4] Typically, a nurse is assigned to review the triggers generated each day. This person can investigate the case—read the chart, talk to the staff, examine the patient—to see if an error or adverse event occurred. If the events are actually in progress, such as sepsis, the nurse can ensure that the appropriate treatment is being instituted.

Sometimes triggers will not necessarily show an error or adverse event but will identify patients who are at higher risk. A forward-thinking hospital might then assign these patients a higher staff ratio, or place them closer to the nursing station, or have a pharmacist review the medications, or arrange for a visiting nurse after discharge. These interventions can decrease future adverse events, which of course is the goal.

---

Many people are looking to artificial intelligence (AI) as a means to decrease medical error and improve patient safety. Eric Topol, a cardiologist in California, probed these issues in his book *Deep Medicine.*[5] AI could be particularly helpful with diagnostic error. As I discussed in chapter 5, AI does especially well with visuals such as chest X-rays and rashes, because you can feed endless images into the system until it learns to recognize patterns and match them to the diagnosis.

Much ink has been spilled about whether AI will surpass doctors in accuracy or even put them out of business altogether. From Topol's perspective, these are the wrong questions to debate. Take the case of skin rashes. Even if AI is no better than a board-certified dermatologist, it could still increase overall diagnostic accuracy because the vast majority of rashes are evaluated and treated by *non*-dermatologists. For all the primary care doctors, nurse practitioners, ER staff, and pediatricians who take care of the majority of skin disease, an AI system could be immensely useful in cutting down diagnostic error.

Topol illustrates a similar situation in ophthalmology. Diabetic retinopathy is one of the leading causes of preventable blindness. Most patients with diabetes do not have their retinopathy diagnosed early enough to prevent visual loss. (A delayed diagnosis falls under the category of diagnostic error.) It's not that ophthalmologists have poor diagnostic skills, but rather that most patients aren't able to get to an eye doctor. As with skin rashes, the key to decreasing overall diagnostic error is to make it possible to get an accurate diagnosis where patients actually are—usually at their family doctor or internist. By feeding hundreds of thousands of retinal images into a computer, there is now an AI algorithm that can make the diagnosis based on a picture taken by a non-ophthalmologist or even a nondoctor. It could be the medical assistant taking the blood pressure who snaps the photo, or even the clerical staff checking in the patient. At some point it could even be the patient taking the picture at home.

But what about diagnosis on a wider scale, something more complex than identifying a clear-cut pattern such as a rash or a retinal picture? When I interviewed Topol, I'd just finished a bruising clinic session that day. My patients came with all sorts of nonspecific complaints—aches, pains, fatigue, dizziness—overlaid upon a flotilla of possibly related or possibly unrelated circumstances—middling triglycerides, "social" alcohol use, a mildly abnormal bone-density scan from six years ago, a cousin with colon cancer, a uric acid level at the upper limits of normal, an EKG with "nonspecific changes," a penchant for McDonald's, a noxious odor at work, gallstones that a doctor thirty years ago mentioned, and so on and so forth. How was AI going to help an internist like me pluck out a correct and actionable diagnosis from the real-world cauldron of confusing possibilities? (And do it while I wrestled with an hour's worth of EMR documentation in the measly fifteen minutes that I was supposed to be using for the history and physical.)

"Well," Topol said, "imagine if you didn't have to chase all of that down. Imagine if the EMR presented you with all the data for the patient—all the scans, all the labs, all the history—all in one place and you didn't have to hunt for everything. And it also had the patient's genome and access to all medical research. And the chart had been edited by the patient for accuracy.

"You wouldn't have to *do* anything," he continued. "You could spend your entire time talking to the patient. The EMR would use 'natural language processing' technology to listen to your conversation and condense it into a concise clinical note. And if you ordered an incorrect or unnecessary test, it would provide you with a reference to explain why you might consider something else."

I had to admit that sounded appealing—using the *entire* visit to interact with the patient rather than with the EMR. That alone would probably decrease my error rate (and my daily spasms of splenic ravings). But I'm especially tantalized by the possibility of AI to cross-connect things that I don't have the bandwidth to keep in my brain—the blood tests from last year, how effective statins are if taken only intermittently, how heritable gastric cancer is, how accurate an MRI is for detecting lymph node disease, the false-positive rate of mammograms in postmenopausal women, which kind of vasculitis affects the intestines, when immunity from the measles vaccine begins to wane, how effective protein restriction is in advanced kidney disease, which rare illnesses arise from the patient's country/city/village of origin, and so on.

Topol's point is not that AI would necessarily be better than me—although it certainly sounds like it has a fighting chance!—but that it could allow me to practice medicine at the top end of my abilities, rather than squandering 97% of my time and focus as a frazzled data-entry clerk. It would allow me to do the things that I'm better at—teasing out a complicated history, picking up on emotional and nonverbal cues, weighing complex treatment options that don't have a right answer, problem-solving the real-world issues that patients face when coping with disease. The other tasks—surveying the 2 million research papers published every year, flipping through the 3,000 pages of my internal medicine textbook, digging through 80,000 bytes of data entered into the EMR per patient per year—could all be left to AI, which can surely do it more comprehensively and more briskly than I can. Without getting a migraine. Or an ulcer. Or carpal tunnel syndrome. Or so burned out that it considers quitting medicine and getting an MBA instead. (Okay, only kidding on that last one . . .)

A major part of tackling medical error is coaxing the issue out of the healthcare world and into the larger society. Patient safety has to permeate the national discourse the way, say, automobile safety did in the 1970s, launching a raft of government regulations and industry initiatives that ultimately led to a precipitous decline in car-related deaths and injuries.

In Denmark, the Patient Safety Act of 2003 led to broader societal changes in how medical error is viewed. In the United States, a Patient Safety Act was passed in 2005, but it was nowhere near as comprehensive as the Danish version. The US law has increased awareness, but it has not initiated a wholesale restructuring of the healthcare and liability systems. Most glaringly, the law did not create any sort of national incident reporting system. This is partly from an American aversion to centralized actions but more practically because no money was allotted to create and administer such a program.

The job of carrying out the Patient Safety Act in the US fell to a small government agency, AHRQ (affectionately called *Arc* by those in the know, but which stands for Agency for Healthcare Research and Quality). AHRQ helps healthcare systems set up their own Patient Safety Organizations (called PSOs in this acronym-addicted field). These PSOs act locally, promoting the voluntary reporting of adverse events. To encourage medical professionals to report, the Patient Safety Act specifies that this information is confidential and cannot be used to discipline the person filing the report. AHRQ manages a network of patient-safety databases, but it doesn't have the resources to integrate everything, nor the teeth to enforce anything.

AHRQ's biggest success is on the educational front. It set up the Patient Safety Network, an online resource that houses a trove of information for the public as well as for medical professionals and administrators. The website (www.psnet.ahrq.gov) offers online learning modules, how-to guides, podcasts, updates about the latest research, and case reports—submitted by the public—that are analyzed by experts. (The cases, by the way, can be submitted anonymously.) The Patient Safety Network attempts to fill the yawning gaps in medical and nursing schools that leave most medical professionals unprepared to recognize, handle, and prevent medical error.

It's not clear if the United States will ever be able to solidify a comprehensive national reporting system, as Denmark has. The closest it has come is in the Veterans Administration (VA) medical system. The VA itself is larger than the entire Danish medical system, but in some ways it has more in common with Danish socialized medicine than the American privatized system. The VA has a single payment system for its more than 1,200 healthcare facilities that cover nearly all the medical needs of veterans. All the facilities use the same EMR, and most of its operational systems are standardized. I once visited a VA hospital in California and everything was eerily identical to our VA hospital in Manhattan, down to the binders for the medical charts, the odd-sized paper they used, and the color scheme of the patients' pajamas.

The VA Patient Safety Reporting System was spearheaded in 1999 by Jim Bagian, a former astronaut who sought to transplant the NASA "systems approach" to healthcare. (The Danish incident reporting system, in fact, is based on this VA reporting system.) Bagian, who is also a physician, argued strongly to shift the focus from "Whose fault is this?" to "What happened, why did it happen, and what can we do to prevent it in the future?"

Importantly, Bagian focused on the reasons that medical professionals don't report errors. "If you ask doctors," he told me, "they'll say it's because they're worried about malpractice." But when the VA did an anonymous survey, the overwhelming reason that doctors did not report errors was because of the profound shame.

When I was a resident, I once botched the diagnosis of an intracranial bleed. Somewhere in the handoff of care, somebody had said, "Radiology fine," and so I hadn't bothered to look at the CT scan myself. I was ready to sashay the patient back home, but luckily the bleed was caught by someone else. The patient went straight to the operating room to have the blood drained from his skull, and he did fine. Technically, my error would be called a "near miss," since the patient's care was ultimately not impacted by my oversight.

But "near miss" hardly captures the essence of what had transpired. "Near miss" just means that the patient got lucky. My error—relying on a verbal report rather than looking at the scan myself—was still an error. I had still put my patient's life at risk. I was so ashamed that I had given substandard care that I did not tell a soul. It took me more than twenty years to talk about it publicly.

At the time, I was so devastated that I could hardly function. As a fledgling physician, I felt that I had failed my patient so gravely that I was ready to quit medicine altogether. I wasn't surprised, years later, to read of a nurse who took her own life after an accidental miscalculation of a medication dose killed an infant in her care.[6]

The famed French surgeon René Leriche wrote, "Every surgeon carries about him a little cemetery, in which from time to time he goes to pray, a cemetery of bitterness and regret, of which he seeks the reason for certain of his failures." This patient with the intracranial bleed resides in my cemetery, as does Ms. Romero—whose anemia and cancer I missed—and, regretfully, many others. Like all doctors and nurses, I visit that cemetery periodically, painfully, even though I'm well aware that the effect of the errors on me is secondary to the effects on the patient. Even with the passage of time and the smoothing over of the graves, the stinging sadness and shame of having harmed your patient never recedes.

This reinforces the bedrock principle that medical error and patient safety issues will never be fully resolved with a blitzkrieg of mandates, checklists, and zero-tolerance policies. The human element is paramount. In fact, Jim Bagian doesn't even use the term "medical error." "The term 'error,'" he wrote to me in an email, "implies a person-centered approach rather than a more effective systems-based approach that includes the person but generally yields solutions that are more sustainable. Experienced safety professionals usually choose the term 'adverse medical events' since you are trying to prevent the event that harms a patient."

Bagian was careful to acknowledge that some situations are indeed "blameworthy." Obvious ones would be when a staff member is inebriated or has committed an actual crime. The other category of blameworthy events would be when a doctor or nurse knowingly and deliberately performs an unsafe action. These events are rare but should be disciplined accordingly. For all the rest, the person who makes the error should take responsibility, but the institutional focus should be on how the system made that error possible and how it could be prevented in the future.

---

When I started writing this book, I set out to determine whether or not medical error truly was the third-leading cause of death, as the headlines had proclaimed. Now that I've spent several years digging through the research and interviewing patients, families, doctors, lawyers, nurses, administrators, researchers, and patient-safety advocates, I've concluded that the question itself isn't as relevant as I'd thought it would be.

In terms of the paper from the *British Medical Journal* that drew this conclusion, there was a fair amount of academic criticism. The first issue was that it wasn't a primary-source study, in which researchers sifted through medical charts trying to figure out whether and where medical errors occurred. Rather, it was a reanalysis of previously published data. The authors certainly didn't present it as anything other than that, but in the public eye it came across as a "brand-new study" that "proved" that medical error was the third leading cause of death. Reanalyzing data, per se, isn't against the rules (the Institute of Medicine used the same technique in its report *To Err Is Human*), but it can introduce flaws and biases. In particular, it is problematic to take results from a narrow slice of life and then extrapolate them to the entire population. Statistically speaking, this is risky business.

For example, one of the four studies the analysis relied upon drew its data from ten hospitals in North Carolina.[7] It's not that these data are necessarily wrong, but they may not accurately represent the entire population. This is particularly precarious when you are dealing with infrequent events. In these ten hospitals, the researchers of this original study concluded that fourteen people died as a result of medical error (out of 2,344 cases reviewed). Fourteen is a very small number. If three more patients had died, the death rate in the study would have jumped up by 20%. When you extrapolate 2,344 cases to a nation of 330 million people, a difference of 20% represents almost a half million extra deaths. So you can see that tiny shifts in a small sample size can exert outsize effects when you try to draw a conclusion about the general population.

Then, of course, there's the challenge of deciding whether an error, in fact, caused the death in question. A patient with end-stage colon cancer may have been given an incorrect medication dose. This is clearly a medical error, but the patient may have died simply from the colon cancer. Parsing causality is not at all straightforward. In the studies upon which the *BMJ* analysis was based, researchers could not always agree whether a particular error caused (or hastened) death. The fourteen deaths due to medical error reported in the North Carolina study might, in reality, have been seventeen deaths, or twelve (which, when extrapolated to the general population and its affection for aviation metaphors, would result in entirely different numbers of jumbo jets crashing). It remains remarkably difficult to calculate precisely how many deaths are caused by medical errors.

When I interviewed Martin Makary, the lead author on the *BMJ* paper, he emphasized that pinpointing *any* cause of death is challenging: "Every cause of death is an estimate. It's not a perfect science." Unfortunately, death certificates require doctors to pick one primary cause of death, which is often impossible. "How do you take a complex series of factors," Makary asked, "and identify a single cause?"

The intense media focus on errors as a "leading cause of death" shifted attention away from all the errors that are happening but *aren't* leading to death (a far larger number). While these errors may not kill patients, they can cause severe harms—amputation, kidney failure, debilitating pain, paralysis, anaphylaxis, financial ruin. These cases won't appear in stats that count only deaths, but they are serious enough to warrant being grouped together in the severe-harms-from-medical-error category when we are trying to assess the overall toll of medical error. And then, of course, there are all the errors that cause no harms at all, which get completely ignored when the focus is solely on the death rate. These smaller errors are equally important to address, because they represent the most extensive pool of harm just waiting to happen.

So it's likely that the "third leading cause of death" claim is not accurate. Medical error probably ranks lower on the list of the things that mow us down. But the fact that it's lower on the list doesn't make the issue any less critical. *Any* harm to patients that is preventable is something we should be aggressively investigating.

My takeaway is that medical error and adverse events (even ones that aren't errors per se) are much more prevalent than we think. The majority may not cause significant harms, but enough do, enough that the issue needs to be front and center in healthcare today. So even if the *BMJ* paper was not correct in its final numbers—numbers which, in any case, may not even be possible to calculate accurately—it did serve to bring public attention to the issue.

Makary pointed out that there is currently no way to indicate medical error on a death certificate. Death certificates are one of the primary ways we collect epidemiological data about the population. That's how we know that heart disease and cancer are the leading causes of death in the United States. (The third leading cause of death, incidentally, is accidents, followed by emphysema and stroke.) Makary proposes that in addition to the standard cause of death, death certificates ought to have an additional field asking whether a preventable complication contributed to the death. This way we might actually know how many errors are occurring—at least those ones that caused or hastened death. As Florence Nightingale pointed out back in 1850, you can't start fixing anything until you gather the data to establish the current state of affairs.

Would doctors actually check such a box? That's a debatable question, given that fear of lawsuits—in the US at least—remains pervasive. But there's

no doubt that we need some sort of unified national database for medical errors, adverse events, and any preventable harm. Mandatory reporting would
likely backfire, and voluntary reporting catches only a small subset of errors.
The only way to make such a system workable and accurate is to create a culture in which reporting an adverse event is a routine and ordinary event for
medical professionals, just like—*ahem*—washing your hands before touching
a patient. Obviously, this would require a culture shift of colossal proportions,
but that is the goal we should be striving toward.

A generation or two ago, the medical system was viewed with unmitigated
reverence. Now the pendulum has swung so far the other way that many
view the medical world with such suspicion that they avoid even routine and
well-validated medical care. The truth settles somewhere in between. Medical science has made enormous strides in the past century and has objectively
decreased mortality and suffering on a grand scale. Our great-grandparents
would give their eyeteeth for the medical benefits that we take for granted today—vaccinations, anesthesia, cancer treatments, heart transplants, dialysis.
But there's no doubt that medical care also causes harm, a good deal of which
is likely preventable. Patients and families—as well as medical staff—should
cast a careful, questioning eye on all medical tests and treatments.

Medicine is a team sport, and that team isn't just the doctors and nurses
but also the patients, families, and closest friends. Too often it can feel like we
are on opposing teams, or at least on teams with opposing agendas. But really,
there is just that one goal: helping the patient get better. There's a plethora of
technology out there to assist the patient in getting better, but the responsibility for making sure it all works falls to the humans.

The IOM certainly picked the title of its groundbreaking report well. To
err is definitely human. It's also human, however, to care about what happens
when error occurs. This holds for the immediate aftermath with an individual
patient, as well as for thinking forward, more broadly, about how to minimize
errors for all patients. We all enter the medical system with the expectation
that we will come out better at the other end or, at least, not worse off. We
certainly have the right to expect that the medical care itself does not make
us worse off. Almost 2,500 years ago, Hippocrates offered some advice to his
fellow Greek healers, writing in his treatise *Of the Epidemics*: "As to diseases,
make a habit of two things—to do good, or at least to do no harm." No one
has said it better since.

# ACKNOWLEDGMENTS

Medical error isn't the most comfortable topic to talk about. Even conscientious and reflective doctors and nurses recoil from dwelling on these lowest moments of their careers. For patients and families, it can be exquisitely painful to recount the details of what robbed them of health, happiness, and life, as well as faith in the medical profession. Thus I have to offer immeasurable gratitude (and credit) to Tara Duke, Melissa Clarkson, and Nancy Clarkson. These three spent hours upon hours sharing their harrowing ordeals, and were extraordinarily generous with their thoughts and feedback. I never had the opportunity to meet Jay or Glenn, but I have been so fortunate for this chance to learn about their jokes, quirks, and loves, in addition to their sobering medical stories. I am honored to have been let into the lives of these two remarkable men.

Many researchers contributed to this book, and I am grateful for the time they took to explain their work. They benevolently answered my dozens of emails and scores of nitpicky questions about their data. An enormous thanks to Hardeep Singh, Mark Graber, Itiel Dror, Bob Wachter, Peter Pronovost, Martin Makary, Thomas Gallagher, Michelle Mello, Eric Topol, and Jim Bagian.

I am indebted to the great Danes who infected me with their enthusiasm and also welcomed me to their country of equally pristine coastlines and bicycle lanes: Louise Rabøl, Beth Lilja, Charlotte Wamberg Rasmussen, Frits Bredal and Martin Erichsen. I confess that whenever I'm feeling overwhelmed in my clinic, I sometime surreptitiously browse one-way airfares to Copenhagen.

Thank you to Ekene Ojukwu, Peter Mullenix, and Elihu Schimmel for sharing their stories. These varied perspectives enriched the book immensely. Jenny Vaughan and Alec Goldenberg generously reviewed some of the medical cases in the book, for which I am so appreciative. I am indebted to Kiran Gupta, who cheerfully ran a fine-toothed, patient-safety comb over the entire manuscript. Her sharp intellect and extensive knowledge of the literature strengthened the book. Many other researchers graciously responded to my cold-call queries, diving into the data with me, sharing resources, directing me to other colleagues. The instinctive openness and intellectual hospitality of the research community never fails to impress me.

Thank you also to Anna Falvey, Briana Crockett, and Katherine Nazzaro for their assistance with initial research forays into the Danish medical system.

I want to give a special shout-out to my colleagues at Bellevue Hospital and NYU School of Medicine, as well as my co-editors at the *Bellevue Literary Review*, for their ongoing support and encouragement. Adina Kalet and Ruth Crowe kindly allowed me to observe their simulation program with medical students and interns. Numerous other colleagues fielded desperate questions, and quite a few magnanimously juggled clinic coverage with me (and occasionally administered Epic CPR) when I was afflicted with cerebral insufficiency. I've been at Bellevue Hospital for more than two decades now, and I can say—without any fear of making a medical error—that it is a singular and stupendous place to work. Bellevue is steeped in history, yet relentlessly modern, reflecting the evolving world with peerless accuracy. There is an unstinting generosity of spirit that encompasses the staff, the patients, and the nearly three centuries of medical care that we share between us. I came to Bellevue as a medical student, cut my teeth as a resident there, and will likely exit only on a gurney. As anyone who has ever worked there can tell you, there is never a dull day at Bellevue. For that I'm ever grateful.

Words cannot fully convey my depth of appreciation to the staff of Beacon Press—though luckily, words are never in short supply in a publishing house. Helene Atwan has been my editor through all of my books, and is the master of amiable but exacting feedback. Her tenacious energy set this book in motion and thankfully didn't let up until the last dangling participle was duly undangled. I am indebted to Pam MacColl and Alyssa Hassan, whose publicity and marketing work are second to none. The magnificent Tom Hallock retired, after twenty-two years at Beacon, and is still sorely missed. A heartfelt thank-you to the entire Beacon production team—Haley Lynch, Susan Lumenello, Marcy Barnes, Louis Roe, Sanj Kharbanda, Christian Coleman, Steven Horne—who transformed this book into an actual book.

Lastly, I want to thank my family. Naava, Noah, and Ariel have all achieved perfectly calibrated teenager ennui, which allows them to effortlessly tune out all parental opinion and advice. Nevertheless, love manages to weave in and out, and I relish every bit. This book is my first without the presence of our dear, sweet Juliet. Seventeen years in dog-years may be close to a century in human years, but it wasn't nearly enough for us. Writing without a warm, black, furry body nestled at your feet just isn't the same.

And thank you, Benjy, for your ever-steadying presence in my life. Decision-making in life—as in medicine—is complicated, fraught with risks and miscalculations. But my decision to be with you remains one of the clearest and best I've ever made. And, happily, that was no error!

# NOTES

## CHAPTER ONE: JUMBO JETS CRASHING

1. M. A. Makary and M. Daniel, "Medical Error—the Third Leading Cause of Death in the US," *British Medical Journal (BMJ)* 353 (2016): 2139–44, www.ncbi.nlm.nih.gov/pubmed /27143499.

2. L. T. Kohn et al., *To Err Is Human: Building a Safer Health System* (Washington, DC: National Academies Press, 2000), www.ncbi.nlm.nih.gov/pubmed/25077248.

3. R. H. Moser, "Diseases of Medical Progress," *New England Journal of Medicine* 255 (1956): 606–14, www.ncbi.nlm.nih.gov/pubmed/13369682.

4. E. M. Schimmel, "The Hazards of Hospitalization," *Annals of Internal Medicine* 60 (1964): 100–110, www.ncbi.nlm.nih.gov/pubmed/12571347.

5. E. M. Schimmel, "The Physician as Pathogen," *Journal of Chronic Diseases* 16 (1963): 1–4, www.ncbi.nlm.nih.gov/pubmed/13991732.

6. T. A. Brennan et al., "Incidence of Adverse Events and Negligence in Hospitalized Patients—Results of the Harvard Medical Practice Study I," *New England Journal of Medicine* 324 (1991): 370–76, www.ncbi.nlm.nih.gov/pubmed/1987460.

7. L. L. Leape, "Error in Medicine," *Journal of the American Medical Association (JAMA)* 272 (1994): 1851–57, www.ncbi.nlm.nih.gov/pubmed/7503827.

8. E. J. Thomas et al., "Incidence and Types of Adverse Events and Negligent Care in Utah and Colorado," *Medical Care* 38 (2000): 261–71, www.ncbi.nlm.nih.gov/pubmed/10718351.

9. S. M. Berenholtz et al., "Eliminating Catheter-Related Bloodstream Infections in the Intensive Care Unit," *Critical Care Medicine* 32 (2004): 2014–20, www.ncbi.nlm.nih.gov /pubmed/15483409.

10. P. J. Pronovost et al., "An Intervention to Decrease Catheter-Related Bloodstream Infections in the ICU," *New England Journal of Medicine* 355 (2006): 2725–32, www.ncbi.nlm .nih.gov/pubmed/17192537.

11. A. B. Haynes, "A Surgical Safety Checklist to Reduce Morbidity and Mortality in a Global Population," *New England Journal of Medicine* 360 (2009): 491–99, www.ncbi.nlm.nih .gov/pubmed/19144931.

12. D. R. Urbach et al., "Introduction of Surgical Safety Checklists in Ontario, Canada," *New England Journal of Medicine* 370 (2014): 1029–38, www.ncbi.nlm.nih.gov/pubmed /24620866.

13. C. Dreifus, "Doctor Leads Quest for Safer Ways to Care for Patients," *New York Times*, March 8, 2010, www.nytimes.com/2010/03/09/science/09conv.html.

14. L. L. Leape, "The Checklist Conundrum," editorial, *New England Journal of Medicine* 370 (2014): 1063–64, www.ncbi.nlm.nih.gov/pubmed/24620871.

15. M. Best and D. Neuhauser, "Ignaz Semmelweis and the Birth of Infection Control," *BMJ Quality & Safety* 13 (2004): 233–34, www.ncbi.nlm.nih.gov/pubmed/15175497.

16. C. J. Gill and G. C. Gill, "Nightingale in Scutari: Her Legacy Reexamined," *Clinical Infectious Diseases* 40 (2005): 1799–1805, www.ncbi.nlm.nih.gov/pubmed/15909269.

### CHAPTER THREE: MAKING—OR MISSING—THE DIAGNOSIS

1. M. L. Graber, "The Incidence of Diagnostic Error in Medicine," *BMJ Quality & Safety* 22 (2013): ii21–ii27, www.ncbi.nlm.nih.gov/pubmed/23771902.

2. H. Singh et al., "Types and Origins of Diagnostic Errors in Primary Care Settings," *JAMA Internal Medicine* 173 (2013): 418–25, www.ncbi.nlm.nih.gov/pubmed/23440149.

3. M. L. Graber et al., "Cognitive Interventions to Reduce Diagnostic Error: A Narrative Review," *BMJ Quality & Safety* 21 (2012): 535–57, www.ncbi.nlm.nih.gov/pubmed/22543420.

### CHAPTER FIVE: DIAGNOSTIC THINKING

1. P. Rajpurkar et al., "Deep Learning for Chest Radiograph Diagnosis: A Retrospective Comparison of the CheXNeXt Algorithm to Practicing Radiologists," *PLoS Medicine* 15, no. 11 (November 20, 2018): e1002686, www.ncbi.nlm.nih.gov/pubmed.

2. N. Riches et al., "The Effectiveness of Electronic Differential Diagnoses (DDX) Generators: A Systematic Review and Meta-Analysis," *PLoS ONE* (March 8, 2016), www.ncbi .nlm.nih.gov/pubmed/26954234.

3. J. W. Ely et al., "Checklists to Reduce Diagnostic Errors," *Academic Medicine* 86 (2011): 307–13, www.ncbi.nlm.nih.gov/pubmed/21248608.

4. Perioperative Interactive Education, "Diagnostic Checklist," Toronto General Hospital, Department of Anesthesia, pie.med.utoronto.ca/DC/DC_content/DC_checklist.html, accessed September 4, 2019.

5. M. L. Graber et al., "Developing Checklists to Prevent Diagnostic Error in Emergency Room Settings," *Diagnosis* (Berl) 1 (2014): 223–31, www.ncbi.nlm.nih.gov/pubmed/27006889.

6. H. Singh and L. Zwaan, "Reducing Diagnostic Error—A New Horizon of Opportunities for Hospital Medicine," *Annals of Internal Medicine* 165 (2016): HO2–HO4, www.ncbi .nlm.nih.gov/pubmed/27750328.

7. E. P. Balogh, B. T. Miller, and J. R. Ball Jr., eds., *Improving Diagnosis in Health Care* (Washington, DC: National Academies Press, 2015), www.ncbi.nlm.nih.gov/books/NBK338600.

### CHAPTER SEVEN: FOR THE RECORD

1. Robert Wachter, *The Digital Doctor: Hope, Hype, and Harm at the Dawn of Medicine's Computer Age* (New York: McGraw Hill, 2015).

2. D. R. Murphy et al., "The Burden of Inbox Notifications in Commercial Electronic Health Records," *JAMA Internal Medicine* 176 (2016): 559–60, www.ncbi.nlm.nih.gov/pubmed/26974737.

3. D. C. Radley et al., "Reduction in Medication Errors in Hospitals Due to Adoption of Computerized Provider Order Entry Systems," *Journal of the American Medical Informatics Association* 20 (2013): 470–76, www.ncbi.nlm.nih.gov/pubmed/23425440.

4. B. J. Drew et al., "Insights into the Problem of Alarm Fatigue with Physiologic Monitor Devices: A Comprehensive Study of Intensive Care Patients," *PLoS One* (October 22, 2014), www.ncbi.nlm.nih.gov/pubmed/25338067.

5. Liz Kowalczyk, "Patient Alarms Often Unheard, Unheeded," *Boston Globe*, February 13, 2011, http://archive.boston.com/lifestyle/health/articles/2011/02/13/patient_alarms_often _unheard_unheeded.

6. M. L. Graber et al., "Electronic Health Record–Related Events in Medical Malpractice Claims," *Journal of Patient Safety* 15 (2019): 77–85, www.ncbi.nlm.nih.gov/pubmed/26558652.

7. "Case Counts," Centers for Disease Control and Prevention, www.cdc.gov/vhf/ebola /outbreaks/2014-west-africa/case-counts.html, accessed December 5, 2019.

8. Josh Vorhees, "Everything That Went Wrong in Dallas," *Slate*, October 16, 2014, http:// www.slate.com/articles/health_and_science/medical_examiner/2014/10/dallas_ebola _timeline_the_many_medical_missteps_at_texas_health_presbyterian.html; D. K. Upadhyay et al., "Ebola US Patient Zero: Lessons on Misdiagnosis and Effective Use of Electronic Health Records," *Diagnosis* 1 (2014): 283–87, www.ncbi.nlm.nih.gov/pubmed/26705511.

9. NBC News, "Texas Hospital Makes Changes after Ebola Patient Turned Away," October 3, 2014, www.nbcnews.com/storyline/ebola-virus-outbreak/texas-hospital-makes-changes -after-ebola-patient-turned-away-n217296.

10. Robert Wachter, "What Ebola Error in Dallas Shows," *USA Today*, October 12, 2014, www.usatoday.com/story/opinion/2014/10/12/what-ebola-error-in-dallas-shows-column /17159839.

## CHAPTER NINE: ON THE CLOCK

1. BBC News, "Leicester Doctor Guilty of Manslaughter of Jack Adcock, 6," November 4, 2015, www.bbc.com/news/uk-england-leicestershire-34722885.

2. *Resident Duty Hours: Enhancing Sleep, Supervision, and Safety* (Washington, DC: National Academies Press, 2009), www.ncbi.nlm.nih.gov/pubmed/25009922.

3. K.Y. Bilimoria et al., "National Cluster-Randomized Trial of Duty-Hour Flexibility in Surgical Training," *New England Journal of Medicine* 374 (2016): 713–27, www.ncbi.nlm.nih .gov/pubmed/26836220.

4. S. Sen et al., "A Prospective Cohort Study Investigating Factors Associated with Depression during Medical Internship," *Archives of General Psychiatry* 67 (2010): 557–65, www.ncbi.nlm.nih.gov/pubmed/20368500; S. C. Fitzgibbons et al., "Long-Term Follow-Up on the Educational Impact of ACGME Duty Hour Limits: A Pre-Post Survey Study," *Annals of Surgery* 256 (2012): 1108–12, www.ncbi.nlm.nih.gov/pubmed/23069864; C. L. Bennett et al., "Association of the 2003 and 2011 ACGME Resident Duty Hour Reforms with Internal Medicine Initial Certification Examination Performance," *Journal of Graduate Medical Education* 9 (2017): 789–90, www.ncbi.nlm.nih.gov/pubmed/29270281.

5. C. P. Landrigan et al., "Effect of Reducing Interns' Work Hours on Serious Medical Errors in Intensive Care Units," *New England Journal of Medicine* 351 (2004): 1838–48, www.ncbi .nlm.nih.gov/pubmed/15509817.

6. J. H. Silber et al., "Patient Safety Outcomes under Flexible and Standard Resident Duty-Hour Rules," *New England Journal of Medicine* 380 (2019): 905–14, www.ncbi.nlm.nih .gov/pubmed/30855740.

7. L. A. Riesenberg et al., "Residents' and Attending Physicians' Handoffs: A Systematic Review of the Literature," *Academic Medicine* 84 (2009): 1775–87, www.ncbi.nlm.nih.gov /pubmed/19940588.

8. A. J. Starmer et al., "Changes in Medical Errors after Implementation of a Handoff Program," *New England Journal of Medicine* 371 (2014): 1803–12, www.ncbi.nlm.nih.gov /pubmed/25372088.

9. D. M. Olds and S. P. Clarke, "The Effect of Work Hours on Adverse Events and Errors in Health Care," *Journal of Safety Research* 41 (2010): 153–62, www.ncbi.nlm.nih.gov/pubmed /20497801.

10. L. H. Aiken et al., "Hospital Nurse Staffing and Patient Mortality, Nurse Burnout, and Job Dissatisfaction," *JAMA* 288 (2002): 1987–93, www.ncbi.nlm.nih.gov/pubmed /12387650.

11. J. Needleman et al., "Nurse Staffing and Inpatient Hospital Mortality," *New England Journal of Medicine* 364 (2011): 1037–45, www.ncbi.nlm.nih.gov/pubmed/21410372.

12. J. Q. Young et al., "July Effect: Impact of the Academic Year-End Changeover on Patient Outcomes: A Systematic Review," *Annals of Internal Medicine* 155 (2011): 309–15, www.ncbi.nlm.nih.gov/pubmed/21747093.

13. L. A. Pauls et al., "The Weekend Effect in Hospitalized Patients: A Meta-Analysis," *Journal of Hospital Medicine* 9 (2017): 760–66, www.ncbi.nlm.nih.gov/pubmed/28914284.

14. A. S. Walker et al., "Mortality Risks Associated with Emergency Admissions during Weekends and Public Holidays: An Analysis of Electronic Health Records," *Lancet* 390 (2017): 62–72, www.ncbi.nlm.nih.gov/pubmed/28499548.

## CHAPTER TEN: WHAT YOU SEE

1. M. F. MacDorman et al., "Trends in Maternal Mortality by Sociodemographic Characteristics and Cause of Death in 27 States and the District of Columbia," *Obstetrics & Gynecology* 129 (2017): 811–18, www.ncbi.nlm.nih.gov/pubmed/28383383.

2. B. D. Smedley, A. Y. Stith, and A. R. Nelson, eds., *Unequal Treatment: Confronting Racial and Ethnic Disparities in Health Care* (Washington, DC: National Academies Press, 2003), www.ncbi.nlm.nih.gov/pubmed/25032386.

3. J. A. Sabin et al., "Physicians' Implicit and Explicit Attitudes about Race by MD Race, Ethnicity, and Gender," *Journal of Health Care for the Poor and Underserved* 20 (2009): 896–913, www.ncbi.nlm.nih.gov/pubmed/19648715.

4. A. R. Green et al., "Implicit Bias among Physicians and Its Prediction of Thrombolysis Decisions for Black and White Patients," *Journal of General Internal Medicine* 9 (2007): 1231–38, www.ncbi.nlm.nih.gov/pubmed/17594129.

5. M. Alsan et. al., "Does Diversity Matter for Health? Experimental Evidence from Oakland," National Bureau of Economic Research Working Paper 24787, revised August 2019, http://www.nber.org/papers/w24787.

6. BBC News, "'Liver Branding' Surgeon Simon Bramhall Fined £10,000," January 12, 2018, www.bbc.com/news/uk-england-birmingham-42663518.

7. Debra Roter and Judith Hall, *Doctors Talking with Patients/Patients Talking with Doctors: Improving Communication in Medical Visits* (Westport, CT: Praeger, 2006), 67–68.

## CHAPTER ELEVEN: I'LL SEE YOU IN COURT

1. T. Halwani and M. Takrouri, "Medical Laws and Ethics of Babylon as Read in Hammurabi's Code," *Internet Journal of Law, Healthcare, and Ethics* 4, no. 2 (2006), ispub.com /IJLHE/4/2/10352.

2. D. P. Kessler, "Evaluating the Medical Malpractice System and Options for Reform," *Journal of Economic Perspectives* 25 (2011): 93–110, www.ncbi.nlm.nih.gov/pubmed/21595327.

3. Carol Peckham, "Medscape Malpractice Report 2015: Why Most Doctors Get Sued," Medscape, December 9, 2015, www.medscape.com/features/slideshow/public/malpractice -report-2015.

4. I. M. Pellino et al., "Consequences of Defensive Medicine, Second Victims, and Clinical-Judicial Syndrome on Surgeons' Medical Practice and on Health Service," *Updates in Surgery* 67 (2015): 331–37, www.ncbi.nlm.nih.gov/m/pubmed/26650202.

5. D. M. Studdert et al., "Claims, Errors, and Compensation Payments in Medical Malpractice Litigation," *New England Journal of Medicine* 354 (2006): 2024–33, www.ncbi.nlm .nih.gov/pubmed/16687715.

## CHAPTER TWELVE: IS THERE A BETTER WAY?

1. M. M. Mello et al., "Administrative Compensation for Medical Injuries: Lessons from Three Foreign Systems," *Commonwealth Fund Issue Brief* 14 (2011): 1–18, www.ncbi.nlm.nih .gov/pubmed/21770079.

2. Olga Pierce and Marshall Allen, "How Denmark Dumped Medical Malpractice and Improved Patient Safety," *ProPublica*, December 31, 2015, www.propublica.org/article/how -denmark-dumped-medical-malpractice-and-improved-patient-safety.

3. Lisa Belkin, "How Can We Save the Next Victim?," *New York Times*, June 15, 1997, www.nytimes.com/1997/06/15/magazine/how-can-we-save-the-next-victim.html.

4. BusinessWire, "Global Dental Floss Market Driven by the Increasing Adoption of Preventive Oral Healthcare Measures, Reports Technavio," April 26, 2017, www.businesswire .com/news/home/20170426006407/en/Global-Dental-Floss-Market-Driven-Increasing -Adoption; Hoosier Econ, "How Much Do Americans Spend on Tattoos?," May 11, 2015, hoosierecon.com/2015/05/11/how-much-do-americans-spend-on-tattoos.

5. P. A. Offit, "Why Are Pharmaceutical Companies Gradually Abandoning Vaccines?," *Health Affairs* 24 (2005): 622–30, www.ncbi.nlm.nih.gov/pubmed/15886152.

6. M. M. Mello et al., "'Health Courts' and Accountability for Patient Safety," *Milbank Quarterly* 84 (2006): 459–92, www.ncbi.nlm.nih.gov/pubmed/16953807.

7. A. Bolton, "Dems Take a Second Look at GOP Proposals, including Tort Reform," *Hill*, February 27, 2010, thehill.com/homenews/house/84021-democrats-take-a-second-look-at-gop-proposals-including-tort-reform.

8. M. M. Mello and A. Kachalia, *Evaluation of Options for Medical Malpractice Reform*, report to the Medicare Payment Advisory Commission (MedPAC), April 2010, http://www.medpac.gov/docs/default-source/reports/dec16_medicalmalpractice_medpac_contractor.pdf.

### CHAPTER THIRTEEN: LOOKING FOR ANSWERS

1. A. C. Mastroianni et al., "The Flaws in State 'Apology' and 'Disclosure' Laws Dilute Their Intended Impact on Malpractice Suits," *Health Affairs* 29 (2010): 1611–19, www.ncbi.nlm.nih.gov/pubmed/20820016.

2. A. Kachalia et al., "Effects of a Communication-and-Resolution Program on Hospitals' Malpractice Claims and Costs," *Health Affairs* 37 (2018): 1836–44, www.ncbi.nlm.nih.gov/pubmed/30395501.

### CHAPTER FOURTEEN: BRINGING ALONG OUR BRAINS

1. I. E. Dror, "A Novel Approach to Minimize Error in the Medical Domain: Cognitive Neuroscientific Insights into Training," *Medical Teacher* 33 (2011): 34–38, www.ncbi.nlm.nih.gov/pubmed/21067318.

2. B. Zendejas et al., "Patient Outcomes in Simulation-Based Medical Education: A Systematic Review," *Journal of General Internal Medicine* 28 (2013): 1078–89, www.ncbi.nlm.nih.gov/pubmed/23595919.

3. J. B. Rousek and M.S. Hallbeck, "Improving Medication Management through the Redesign of the Hospital Code Cart Medication Drawer," *Human Factors* 53 (2011): 626–36, www.ncbi.nlm.nih.gov/pubmed/22235525.

### CHAPTER FIFTEEN: THE RECKONING

1. E. S. Berner and M. L. Graber, "Overconfidence as a Cause of Diagnostic Error in Medicine," *American Journal of Medicine* 121 (2008): S2–S23, www.ncbi.nlm.nih.gov/pubmed/18440350.

### CHAPTER SEVENTEEN: GETTING IT RIGHT

1. J. Arimura et al., "Neonatal Heparin Overdose—A Multidisciplinary Team Approach to Medication Error Prevention," *Journal of Pediatric Pharmacology and Therapeutics* 13 (2008): 96–98, www.ncbi.nlm.nih.gov/pubmed/23055872.

2. C. P. Thirukumaran et al., "Impact of Medicare's Nonpayment Program on Hospital-Acquired Conditions," *Medical Care* 55 (2017): 447–55, www.ncbi.nlm.nih.gov/pubmed/27922910.

3. S. G. Murray et al., "Using Spatial and Temporal Mapping to Identify Nosocomial Disease Transmission of *Clostridium difficile*," *JAMA Internal Medicine* 177 (2017): 1863–65, www.ncbi.nlm.nih.gov/pubmed/29059280.

4. D. Classen et al., "An Electronic Health Record-Based Real-Time Analytics Program for Patient Safety Surveillance and Improvement," *Health Affairs* 37 (2018): 1805–12, www.ncbi.nlm.nih.gov/pubmed/30395491.

5. Eric Topol, *Deep Medicine: How Artificial Intelligence Can Make Healthcare Human Again* (New York: Basic Books, 2019).

6. NBC News, "Nurse's Suicide Highlights Twin Tragedies of Medical Errors," June 27, 2011, http://www.nbcnews.com/id/43529641/ns/health-health_care/t/nurses-suicide-highlights -twin-tragedies-medical-errors.

7 C. P. Landrigan et al., "Temporal Trends in Rates of Patient Harm Resulting from Medical Care," *New England Journal of Medicine* 363 (2010): 2124–34, www.ncbi.nlm.nih.gov /pubmed/21105794.

# INDEX

abdominal pain, differential diagnosis of, 40–42
ACE inhibitors, 62
acute myeloid leukemia (AML), 24–25
acute promyelocytic leukemia (APML), 27
acute respiratory distress syndrome (ARDS), 73, 201–2
Adcock, Jack (child with Down's syndrome), 111–16, 124, 128, 132–33, 143, 181, 197
adrenal insufficiency, diagnosis of, 65–67
adverse events: appropriate responses to, 228–29; Bagian on, 241; definition of, in Harvard Medical Practice Study, 5; internal reviews of, 172; reporting of, 235, 244; as result of handoffs, 120–23. See also medical error
Affordable Care Act (2010), 161–62
Agency for Healthcare Research and Quality (AHRQ), 239–40
(AI) artificial intelligence, 57–59, 128, 237–39
AIDS, harm reduction strategies and, 221
airway protection, in burn treatment, 167
alarms, from medical monitoring devices, prevalence of, 90–92
alerts, EMRs and alert fatigue, 87–92, 101
altruism, in professions, 145
alveoli (air sacs), 73
American Association for Justice (Association of Trial Lawyers of America), 161–62
American Burn Society, transfer criteria for burn victims, 170
American Medical Association, formation of, 136
Amir, Dr. (heme-onc fellow), 30, 51, 71–72, 73, 201–2
AML (acute myeloid leukemia), 24–25
amyloidosis, 62
anemia, diagnosis of, 35–36, 37–38
anesthesia, 176–77, 195, 231
Annals of Internal Medicine, Schimmel article in, 4
APML (acute promyelocytic leukemia), 27

ARDS (acute respiratory distress syndrome), 73
artificial intelligence (AI), 57–59, 128, 237–39
Association of Trial Lawyers of America (American Association for Justice), 161–62
asthma, 62
atelectasis, 75
attending physicians: impact of work rules changes on, 124; July effect and, 126; in digoxin overdose case, 154; responsibilities of, 54, 116; senior doctors as, 111; simulations and, 194; in Zion case, 115. See also McAuliffe, Vincent; Mueller, Dr.
autologous bone marrow transplants, 25
autopsies, decline in numbers of, 40
aviation industry, 8–9, 64–65, 220

Bactrim (antibiotic), 85–87
Bagian, Jim, 240, 241
Bawa-Garba, Hadiza (pediatrics ward registrar), 111–16, 124, 132–33, 143, 181
Bell Commission, 116
Bellevue Hospital: attending physicians, scheduling of, 124; Ebola preparations at, 94; MERS response test, 96–97; work schedule changes at, 119–21. See also Ofri, Danielle
Benadryl (diphenhydramine), 236
bias. See racial bias
BiPAP (breathing mask), 75–76
blame, 134, 241
blood clots in lungs, 62, 207
blood draws, proper procedures for, 198
blood vessels, impact of burns on, 167, 175–76
BMTUs (bone marrow transplant units), 30, 51, 147–49, 202–4, 209
bone marrow biopsies, 22–24
bone marrow transplants, 25, 149
bone marrow transplant units (BMTUs), 30, 51, 147–49, 202–4, 209
Boston Globe, on alarm fatigue deaths, 91
brain: brain-friendly EMR, 185–86; brain-friendly technology, 195; brain-friendly